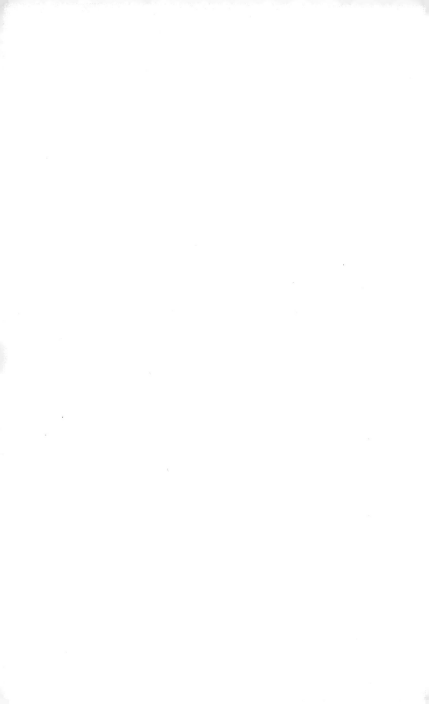

LECTURE NOTES ON
THE INFECTIOUS DISEASES

LECTURE NOTES ON

The Infectious Diseases

JOHN F. WARIN
OBE, MA(Oxon), MD, FRCP, FFCM, DPH
Honorary Consultant in Infectious Diseases
Oxfordshire Area Health Authority (T)

ALASTAIR G. IRONSIDE
MB, ChB, FRCP(Ed)
Consultant Physician
Regional Department of Infectious Diseases
Monsall Hospital, Manchester
Lecturer in Communicable Diseases
University of Manchester

BIBHAT K. MANDAL
MBBS, FRCP(Ed and Glas)
Consultant Physician
Regional Department of Infectious Diseases
Monsall Hospital, Manchester
Lecturer in Communicable Diseases
University of Manchester

THIRD EDITION

BLACKWELL SCIENTIFIC PUBLICATIONS
OXFORD   LONDON   EDINBURGH
BOSTON   MELBOURNE

© 1969, 1974, 1980 by
Blackwell Scientific Publications
Editorial offices:
Osney Mead, Oxford, OX2 0EL
8 John Street, London, WC1N 2ES
9 Forrest Road, Edinburgh, EH1 2QH
52 Beacon Street, Boston, Mass., U.S.A.
214 Berkeley Street, Carlton
   Victoria 3053, Australia

First published 1969
Second edition 1974
Revised reprint 1975
Third edition 1980

Printed in Great Britain by
BELL AND BAIN LTD., GLASGOW
and bound by
KEMP HALL BINDERY, OXFORD

DISTRIBUTORS
USA
   Blackwell Mosby Book Distributors
   11830 Westline Industrial Drive,
   St Louis, Missouri 63141

Canada
   Blackwell Mosby Book Distributors
   86 Northline Road, Toronto,
   Ontario, M4B 3E5

Australia
   Blackwell Scientific Book Distributors
   214 Berkeley Street, Carlton,
   Victoria 3055

British Library
Cataloguing in Publication Data

Warin, John Fairbairn
   Lecture notes on the infectious diseases.
   —3rd ed.
   1. Communicable diseases
   I. Title, II. Ironside, Alastair Grant
   III. Mandal, Bibhat K
   616.9   RC111

   ISBN 0-632-00565-3

Contents

Preface to Third Edition

To write a textbook and to revise it completely three times in ten years is no small undertaking. However in this third edition, a third author (B.K.M.) has brought welcome new ideas and energy to the task. In the four years since the last edition of the book there have been many changes in the field of infectious diseases and a substantial revision has been necessary.

Following adverse publicity about whooping cough vaccine, there has been a disturbing fall in the acceptance rates of all routine infant vaccinations in recent years. Whatever the final outcome of the whooping cough vaccine controversy, it is of great importance that diphtheria, tetanus, poliomyelitis and measles vaccinations should be maintained at a high level.

The discovery of major new antibiotics seems increasingly unlikely. However, refinements of existing drugs continue to appear and while some of these are little more than a change in name, others show increased effectiveness or an improved antibacterial spectrum. There has been as yet no major break-through in antiviral chemotherapy, although new compounds with long names but limited clinical value continue to appear.

Importations of tropical infections are increasing in frequency and variety, for example malaria in Britain has increased more than tenfold in the last few years. It is accepted that infectious diseases departments have the expertise and facilities to deal with the bulk of these tropical infections while a number of the larger departments now provide secure isolation facilities for the more dangerous imported infections.

A number of new conditions are described in this edition, including campylobacter enteritis, clostridial pseudo-membranous colitis, infant botulism, legionnaires disease, Lassa fever and the other viral haemorrhagic fevers. There is a new chapter on worm infections and expanded sections on other conditions such as rabies.

The aim of the book is to provide a concise but fairly full account of infectious diseases practice in this country, for the benefit of medical students and young doctors in hospital, general practice and community medicine.

We would like to thank our secretaries Miss G. Marshall,

Miss R. Allen and Miss M. V. Crabb for undertaking so willingly and expertly the clerical work involved in this Third Edition and also Professor W. Kershaw for his helpful advice on tropical conditions.

J. F. Warin
A. G. Ironside
B. K. Mandal

Colour Plates

We are indebted to Boehringer Ingleheim for their donation of the plates for this section. The original photographs are from the collection of the Regional Department of Infectious Diseases, Monsall Hospital.

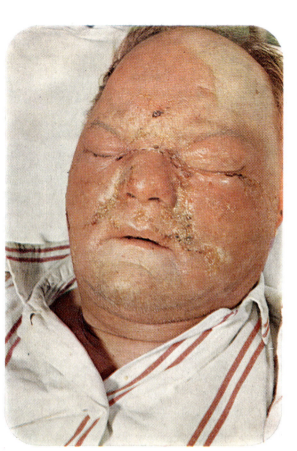

PLATE 1 Erysipelas of the Face.

Showing a raised plaque of erythema with a clear line of demarcation on the forehead. There are superficial vesicles and crusting in the flexures and oedema of the eyelids and nose.

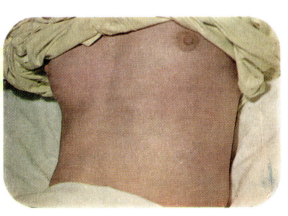

PLATE 2 Scarlet Fever.

Showing a punctate erythema which is a diffuse 'blush' of the skin with a fine stippling of deeper red points.

PLATE 3 Measles (2nd day rash).

Showing a bright generalized maculopapular erythema, confluent over large areas of face, trunk and limbs.

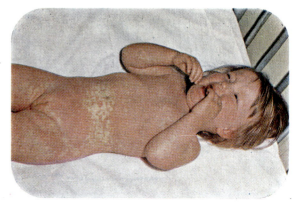

PLATE 4 Measles (5th day rash).

Showing dull, brownish-purple 'staining' of the rash, due to diapedesis of red cells.

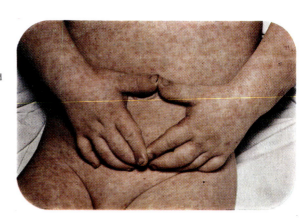

PLATE 5 Toxic Epidermal Necrolysis (also called Ritter's Disease).

Showing the typical 'wet tissue-paper' desquamation on the trunk.

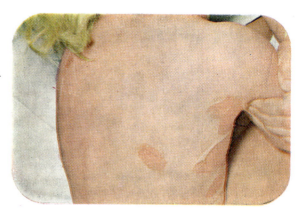

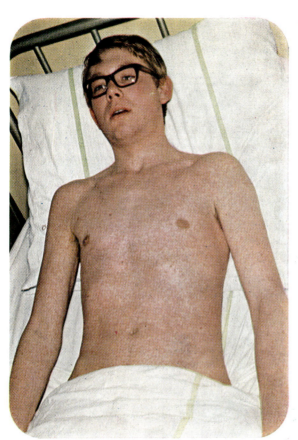

PLATE 6 **Rubella.**
Showing a generalized
discrete macular
erythema.

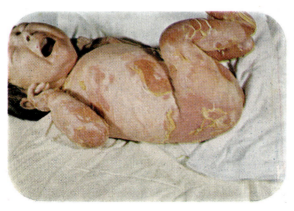

PLATE 7 **Toxic Epi-
dermal Necrolysis**
(formerly called
'pemphigus neonatorum'
in this age group).

Showing widespread
superficial desquamation
leaving a raw inflamed
base.

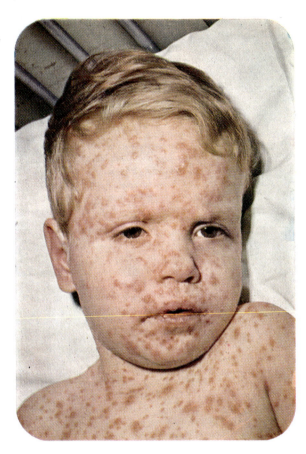

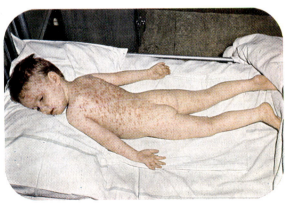

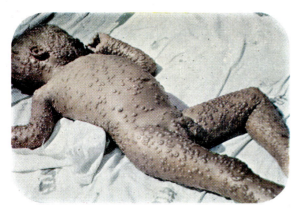

PLATE 10 Smallpox.

Showing large uniform pustules, some umbilicated, with the typical peripheral distribution, most dense on the face and limbs.

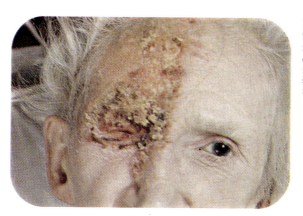

PLATE 11 Herpes Zoster (ophthalmic).

Showing late confluent crusting on the forehead, involving the eye, with sharp demarcation in the midline.

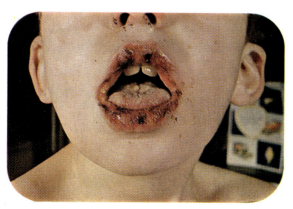

PLATE 12 Herpes Simplex.

Showing primary stomatitis with irregular ulceration of the lips and tongue, and skin vesicles at the left corner of the mouth.

PLATE 13 Cutaneous Anthrax.

Showing an early dark vesicular lesion on the forehead, with oedema of the eyelids.

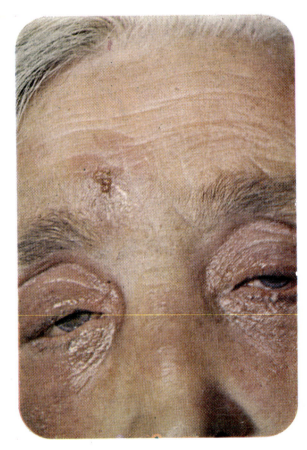

PLATE 14 Meningococcal Meningitis.

Showing irregular scattered petechiae and a few larger purpuric areas.

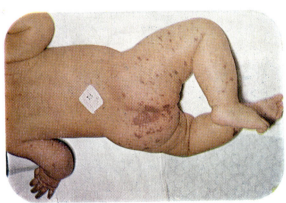

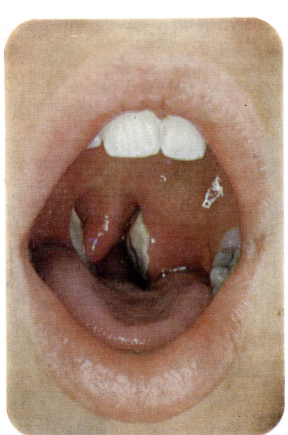

PLATE 15 **Anginose Glandular Fever.**

Showing severe inflammation and oedema of the fauces, with thick creamy membrane over the tonsils.

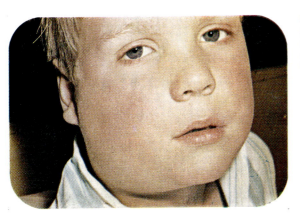

PLATE 16 **Mumps.**

Showing diffuse swelling of the right parotid, obscuring the angle of the jaw.

PLATE 17 Dehydration in Gastroenteritis.

Showing sunken black-ringed eyes and prominence of the skull bones. There is also tissue wasting of the trunk and limbs.

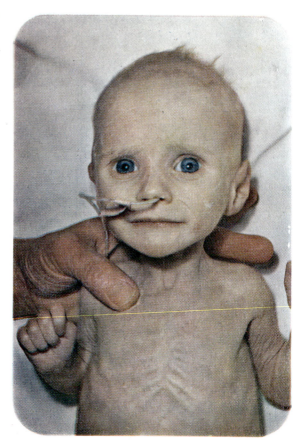

PLATE 18 Typhoid Fever.

Showing sparse periumbilical macules, the 'rose spots'. (Both the typhoid and the suntan were acquired on a Mediterranean holiday.)

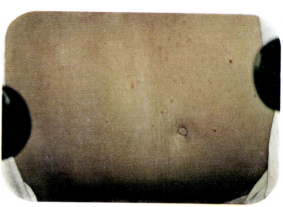

Preface to First Edition

This book is based on lecture notes started by J.F.W. in 1946 for the benefit of medical students at Leeds University. They have been progressively expanded and frequently revised during the last twenty years for the use of medical students in the University of Oxford.

In recent years A.G.I. has assisted in the revision of the lecture notes, and this collaboration has continued throughout the complete rewriting which has been required for publication. It was Oxford medical students who suggested that the lecture notes should be published in book form, and it is primarily for medical students that the book is intended. However, it is hoped that it might also be of help to recently-qualified doctors, whether in hospital or in community practice. Most of the infectious diseases encountered in this country at the present time (including those imported from abroad) have been described.

The authors would like to thank Dr Kathleen Warin of Oxford and Drs Heyworth and Tuxford of Manchester for many helpful suggestions in the preparation of the text, and their secretaries, Miss M. V. Crabb and Miss B. Sherwin, for their most generous response to the extra work involved in the preparation of the typescript.

J.F.W.
A.G.I.

March 1969

CHAPTER 1

Introduction

There has been a spectacular decline in the incidence and mortality of infectious diseases in this country during the last half century, largely due to effective preventive measures. This favourable position can only be maintained or improved upon by the application of measures based on a sound knowledge of these diseases.

Changing patterns of disease
During the last hundred years, there have been many environmental improvements in the developed countries of the world. These have included the provision of pure water supplies and the safe sanitary disposal of excreta, improvements in food and milk hygiene, refuse disposal and the control of insects, lice and rodents. During the same period there has been a great improvement in the nutrition of the population and in the development of health services, with the production of successful vaccines and effective antimicrobial drugs. These measures have led to the virtual disappearance of diseases such as plague, cholera, typhus, smallpox, diphtheria and poliomyelitis, and to a great reduction in others such as tuberculosis, typhoid, whooping cough and more recently measles. Some organisms have become less virulent and this is particularly true of the haemolytic streptococcus which now causes very mild disease compared with that of a hundred years ago.

However, a densely populated country like Britain is still prone to epidemics of influenza and other respiratory virus infections. 'Mass production' farming methods and an increase in communal eating have led to an increase in salmonellosis, while dysentery, infantile gastroenteritis and viral hepatitis remain common diseases. Infections of the nervous system such as bacterial meningitis, viral encephalitis and polyneuritis are uncommon but serious diseases. The venereal infection, gonorrhoea, has greatly increased in incidence over the last decade.

In recent times, the increasing volume and rapidity of foreign travel has led to importations of many exotic diseases, a trend which will undoubtedly increase in the future. In the under-developed countries of the world, particularly in the tropics, infectious disease remains a huge problem with a high mortality. It is accepted that drug treatments and even vaccination pro-grammes make little impact on the problem while the underly-ing factors of poverty, malnutrition and the absence of basic hygienic facilities (such as safe water supply) remain.

Hospitals are dangerous places, prone to outbreaks of in-fection of many kinds. Advances in medical technology such as renal dialysis, the use of immunosuppressive drugs and organ transplants have led to new types of 'opportunist' infection with otherwise harmless micro-organisms.

Table 1 shows the change in incidence and mortality in some of the more important notifiable diseases in England and Wales between 1930 and 1970.

TABLE 1

Disease	1930		1970	
	Notifications	Deaths	Notifications	Deaths
Scarlet Fever	111 077	740	13 138	0
Diphtheria	73 953	3497	22	3
Measles	—	4188	307 279	42
Whooping Cough	—	2037	16 597	15
Smallpox	11 839	28	0	0
Poliomyelitis	591	164	7	0
Meningococcal Infection	664	632	525	143
Typhoid and Paratyphoid	2952	313	368	4
Dysentery	538	97	10 767	7

Host–parasite interaction

Whether or not infection by a pathogenic organism will result in disease and, if so, its severity, depends both on the organism and on the patient.

The factors concerning the organism are its virulence, the dose and the site of infection.

The factors concerning the patient are general health and specific immunity. Adverse factors in the former include fatigue, malnutrition, chronic illness and treatment with immunosuppressive drugs. The very old and the very young usually tolerate infection badly. Specific immunity possessed by the mother is generally passed on as antibody across the placenta to the infant and gives protection during the early and vulnerable months of life; whooping cough is a notable exception. This passive immunity disappears by the age of nine months; thereafter active and lasting protection is obtained by prophylactic immunization or by natural infection.

When infection occurs, the result may be:
1 a typical attack of the illness,
2 a mild illness with indefinite symptoms,
3 no illness at all.

Sources of infection
The source of all human infections may be traced to a human case or carrier or to an animal ranging from insect to mammal. In some cases, there may be a long interval of time between the original excretion of the organism and infection in the new host, particularly with spore-forming infections such as tetanus or anthrax. In certain 'opportunist' infections the source is often the patient's own microbiological flora.

Transmission of infection
Infection spreads by one of the following major methods.

1   Airborne
Infection is exhaled from the case or carrier by coughing, sneezing, speaking or even quiet breathing and is carried by air currents in invisible droplets of moisture which are inhaled by the new host. The droplets may adhere to dust or textiles, when the water evaporates, leaving infected dust which may still transmit infection by air currents for as long as the organism survives.
Diseases spread by the airborne route include:
  (a) *Exanthemata* (diseases characterized by a distinctive rash)—measles, rubella, chickenpox, smallpox, scarlet fever.
  (b) *Mouth and throat infections*—diphtheria, tonsillitis, mumps, herpes stomatitis.

(c) *Respiratory tract infections*—whooping cough, pulmonary tuberculosis, influenza and other respiratory virus infections.

(d) *General*—meningococcal and staphylococcal infection.

2   Intestinal

Infection present in the bowel excreta of a case or carrier is ingested by a fresh host. Transmission may be immediate and direct via infected fingers, eating utensils, clothing, toilets, etc., or indirectly via food or water, where the organism in some cases undergoes a further period of multiplication.

Diseases spread by the intestinal route include typhoid and paratyphoid, salmonellosis, dysentery, cholera, gastroenteritis, viral hepatitis, poliomyelitis and other enterovirus infections.

In another group of zoonotic diseases, transmission is by ingestion of animal flesh or milk. This group includes brucellosis, Q fever, salmonellosis, trichiniasis and other helminth infections.

3 Direct contact

Infection may be transmitted directly by local skin contact. These are mostly cutaneous infections and include impetigo, scabies, cowpox, vaccinia and anthrax.

4   Venereal route

Infection may be transmitted by sexual contact, including syphilis, gonorrhoea, lymphogranuloma venereum, hepatitis B and herpes genitalis infection.

5   Insect or animal bite

Infections transmitted by bites include malaria, trypanosomiasis, typhus, rabies and herpesvirus simiae infection.

These do not cover all the complex routes by which disease spreads. For example, leptospirae excreted in rat's urine may contaminate stagnant water and later penetrate the intact skin of a human host bathing in the water, or tetanus spores from the faeces of herbivorous animals may contaminate pasture land and years later may enter a wound and cause human disease.

Other diseases may spread by two or more alternative routes, for example, tuberculosis commonly spreads by airborne infection, but may spread via milk by ingestion or even by direct skin contact.

Portal of entry

Infection may enter the human host at the following main sites

1 Respiratory tract—airborne infections normally enter by the upper respiratory or occasionally the lower respiratory tracts. The lymphoid tissue of the pharynx is the main localizing site of entry. Once established in the respiratory tract, infection may remain localized (whooping cough), may elaborate an exotoxin which affects distant tissues (diphtheria, scarlet fever) or may disseminate throughout the body (measles, chickenpox).

2 Gastrointestinal tract—intestinal infections mainly localize in the lymphoid tissue of the gastrointestinal tract. Once established, infection may remain localized in the bowel (gastroenteritis, dysentery, salmonellosis) or may disseminate throughout the body (typhoid, brucellosis, Q fever) or rarely may produce distant toxic effects (botulism).

3 The skin—infection may enter the host in several ways via the skin, and may produce localized, generalized or toxic effects.

(a) Direct infection of the skin surface (vaccinia, scabies, impetigo).

(b) Penetration of intact skin (leptospirosis, erysipelas).

(c) Infection of broken skin (wound infections, burn sepsis, tetanus).

(d) Penetration of skin by bites (malaria, typhus, plague, rabies).

(e) Injection through the skin (virus B hepatitis, septicaemia).

Incubation and prodromal periods

These may be of some diagnostic importance.

The *incubation period* is the interval between the time of infection and the first appearance of symptoms of the disease. The incubation period for a disease varies in different patients within an accepted range. They may be grouped in some of the commoner infections as follows:

1 *Short incubation period (up to 1 week)*—scarlet fever, diphtheria, influenza, meningococcal infection, dysentery, gastroenteritis of infancy.

2 *Incubation period 1–2 weeks*—measles, smallpox, whooping cough, poliomyelitis, typhoid.

3 *Incubation period 2–3 weeks*—rubella, chickenpox, mumps.

4 *Incubation period over 3 weeks*—hepatitis A (2–6 weeks), hepatitis B (2–6 months), rabies (4 weeks–1 year or longer).

The *prodromal period* is the interval between the onset of the first symptom and the appearance of the typical rash; it is of value in distinguishing the following:

1   Measles (3–7 days), rubella (0–2 days).
2   Smallpox (2–5 days), chickenpox (0–2 days).

Infectious disease services

The general practitioner undertakes the primary care of all domiciliary cases. He may obtain clinical advice from infectious diseases or other consultants in the hospital service; laboratory assistance from the Public Health Laboratory Service, and epidemiological help from the Medical Officer for Environmental Health (MOEH), who has the ultimate responsibility for community safety in serious infectious diseases.

1   The future planning of hospital services provides for a major infectious diseases department for children and adults in each region, with special facilities for patients and with teaching and research functions. Several of the larger regional units now provide high security isolation facilities capable of dealing with the more dangerous imported diseases such as Lassa Fever. In addition there may be small isolation units in the district general hospital network. In infectious diseases units, the staff are fully immunized and have the expertise and facilities to ensure the safe handling, feeding and treatment of patients and also the safe disposal of crockery, soiled linen and excreta. When a patient is discharged the cubicle is disinfected, the floor, walls and fittings with phenolic disinfectants, and rubber, plastic or wooden articles with hypochlorite solution. Bedding and other textiles are changed and laundered. Normal hospital visiting is allowed, provided the necessary precautions are taken. Mothers are particularly encouraged to visit their children and to play a part in their care. A few small hospitals are maintained exclusively for smallpox cases.

2   The Public Health Laboratory Service (PHLS) maintains a chain of laboratories throughout England and Wales, supported by reference laboratories in London, which provide a diagnostic microbiology service and epidemiological help. The Communicable Diseases Surveillance Centre is a branch of the PHLS responsible for providing information through weekly Communicable Disease Reports and for supporting environmental health staff in serious infections.

3   The Medical Officer of Environmental Health in each Area Health Authority with the support of local authority Environmental Health Officers is responsible for the local control of communicable diseases.
4   The Department of Health and Social Security maintains a communicable diseases section for central policy making including vaccination programmes and international problems.

Control measures
1   Notification
This dates from 1899, and the following is the revised list under the *Public Health (Infectious Diseases) Regulations 1968:*
Anthrax
Cholera
Diphtheria
Dysentery (amoebic or bacillary)
Acute encephalitis (post-infectious or primary)
Food poisoning (including salmonellosis)
Infective jaundice
Leprosy
Leptospirosis
Malaria (recording country of origin)
Measles
Acute meningitis (recording causal organism if known)
Ophthalmia neonatorum (purulent discharge from the eyes of
   an infant commencing within 21 days of birth)
Plague
Acute poliomyelitis (paralytic or non-paralytic)
Relapsing fever
Scarlet fever
Smallpox
Tetanus
Tuberculosis (recording organ or system involved)
Typhoid and paratyphoid fevers
Typhus fever
Whooping cough
Yellow fever

More recently rabies, Lassa fever and Marburg disease have been added to the notifiable diseases list.

The law requires the doctor in attendance on the patient to notify the Medical Officer for Environmental Health of the district in which the patient is living as soon as the diagnosis is made. Notification forms are provided by the local authority, and a doctor is paid a fee for each notification. A local authority may make additional diseases notifiable in its own district; for instance, rubella and glandular fever.

Prompt notification enables the MOEH to instigate control measures where there is serious disease and also provides a valuable record of incidence. The Public Health Laboratory and other hospital laboratories are further important sources of information, from microbiological isolations. Other sources of information include 'spotter' general practitioners who report weekly the incidence of several infections, and occasionally reports from nurseries and schools.

2 Environmental health action

Serious infectious disease cases are investigated by the MOEH, usually in collaboration with infectious diseases and Public Health Laboratory consultants. The source of infection, mode of spread, contacts and occupational circumstances are all investigated and appropriate measures carried out, including the isolation and treatment of patients and the immunization and control of carriers and contacts.

Isolation of patients

The majority of patients are isolated and treated at home. Admission to an infectious diseases unit is requested in the following circumstances;

(a) Patients with severe or complicated infections who require special medical and nursing care, and hospital diagnostic facilities.

(b) Patients presenting with certain features which make them unsafe for admission to general units, e.g. acute diarrhoea, fever or skin rashes; particularly when the disease has originated abroad.

(c) Patients with ordinary infections whose home circumstances make adequate care impossible, e.g. children from seriously overcrowded homes, students in 'digs', hotel guests etc.

(d) Patients with infections dangerous to the community:

   (i) diphtheria cases and carriers,

   (ii) poliomyelitis,

   (iii) typhoid and paratyphoid cases and carriers,

(iv) 'open' tuberculosis (to chest or tuberculosis units),
(v) suspected smallpox or imported viral haemorrhagic disease. (After initial assessment at home, such cases may be admitted to special smallpox hospitals or to secure isolation units.)

Power of compulsory removal to hospital exists, but is rarely used. The discharge of patients from hospital is largely dependent on clinical recovery and it is rarely necessary to continue the treatment of carriers or excretors in hospital, except in severe infections such as diphtheria or typhoid, or where social conditions are highly unsatisfactory.

Control of contacts. Contacts may require daily surveillance, as in smallpox, or they may be excluded from work or school as in typhoid, diphtheria, and poliomyelitis. In these infections, contacts are excluded for the upper limit of the incubation period. Exclusion from work also depends, on the type of employment, so that hospital nurses or food handlers may be excluded in the case of less serious diseases, e.g. salmonellosis.

The practice of exclusion of contacts from school varies in different areas but is becoming less rigid. There is no reason for the routine exclusion of contacts of chickenpox, sonne dysentery, measles, mumps, rubella, scarlet fever and whooping cough, although this may be necessary in certain circumstances, on the advice of the general practitioner or the Specialist in Community Medicine (Child Health).

Control of carriers. Laboratory investigations may detect carriers and mild cases which are possible sources of further infection, and these may be excluded for a time from work or school. There are compulsory powers (*Public Health (Infectious Diseases) Regulations 1968*) to prevent any case or carrier of typhoid, paratyphoid, salmonella infection, amoebic or bacillary dysentery or staphylococcal infection from entering or continuing any occupation connected with food. It may be possible to find alternative and safe employment for such persons but if excluded from work they are entitled to full salary.

International control measures

In cases of smallpox, cholera, plague and yellow fever (officially referred to as 'diseases subject subject to the regulations') the World Health Organization arranges an interchange of information to enable the necessary public health and preventive measures to be carried out. The World Health Organization also regularly exchanges information on a further group of infections which are kept under surveillance and this includes poliomyelitis, epidemic influenza, viral haemorrhagic fevers, louse-borne relapsing and typhus fevers.

CHAPTER 2

Immunization

1   Routine immunization in childhood

In 1978, the Department of Health and Social Security recommended a revised schedule of immunization. The schedule and accompanying notes are shown below (Table 2). One main change in the new schedule is the start at the earlier age of three months to provide protection against whooping cough in younger children. However, it should be pointed out that the main mortality in whooping cough occurs in infants under 6 months of age, so that no schedule of immunization can give complete protection to the most vulnerable age group. It is further suggested that the schedule might be varied in years of high whooping cough incidence, but, unless adopted on a rigid national timetable, this might lead to considerable administrative problems, particularly for children who have moved from one area to another during the schedule. A welcome feature of the new schedule is the extension to include adult life. The Department of Health has now agreed that compensation will be paid to individuals who sustain serious health damage from a recommended routine vaccination.

TABLE 2

Revised schedule 1978

Age	Vaccine	Interval	Notes
During the first year of life	DTPer/Vac/Ads and oral polio vaccine. (1st dose) DTPer/Vac/Ads and oral polio vaccine. (2nd dose) DTPer/Vac/Ads and oral polio vaccine. (3rd dose)	Preferably after an interval of 6–8 weeks Preferably after an interval of 4–6 months	The first dose of triple vaccine (DTPer/Vac/Ads) together with oral poliomyelitis vaccine (Pol/Vac/(Oral)) should be given at 3 months of age. If pertussis vaccine is contra-indicated or declined by the parent diphtheria/tetanus vaccine (DT/Vac/Ads/ should be given. (See additional note 6)
During the second year of life	Measles vaccine	After an interval of not less than 3 weeks following another live vaccine (See additional note 7)	(See additional note 3)
At school entry or entry to nursery school	DT/Vac/Ads and oral polio vaccine	It is preferable to allow an interval of at least 3 years after completing the basic course (See additional note 2)	(See additional note 7)
Between 11 and 13 years of age	BCG vaccine	There should be an interval of not less than 3 weeks between BCG and rubella vaccination (See additional notes 4 & 7)	For tuberculin-negative children. For tuberculin-negative contacts at any age (See additional note 4)

11

Table 2 (*contd.*)   Revised schedule 1978

Age	Vaccine	Interval	Notes
Between 11 and 13 years of age	Rubella vaccine Girls only		All girls of this age should be offered rubella vaccine whether or not there is a past history of an attack of rubella (See additional note 5)
On leaving school or before employment or entering further education	Polio vaccine (oral or inactivated) and tetanus vaccine (Tet/Vac/Ads)	(See additional note 2)	
Adult life	Polio vaccine (oral or inactivated) for previously unvaccinated adults.	A course for previously unvaccinated adults consists of: Oral polio vaccine: three doses with an interval of 6–8 weeks between the first and second doses and of 4–6 months between the second and third: or; Inactivated vaccine: two doses at intervals of 6–8 weeks followed by a third dose 4–6 months later.	For travellers to countries where poliomyelitis is endemic. Unvaccinated parents of a child being given oral polio vaccine should also be offered a course of oral polio vaccine.

TABLE 2 (*contd.*)   Revised schedule 1978

Age	Vaccine	Interval	Notes
Adult life	Rubella vaccine for susceptible women of child-bearing age.	(See additional notes 5 & 7)	Adult females of child-bearing age should be tested for rubella antibodies. Sero-negative women should be offered rubella vaccination. Pregnancy must be excluded before vaccination and the patient must be warned not to become pregnant for 8 weeks after immunization.
	Active immunization against tetanus (Tet/Vac/Ads) for previously unvaccinated adults.	A course for previously unvaccinated adults consists of three doses with an interval of 6–8 weeks between the first and second dose followed by a third dose 6 months later.	

Revised Schedule 1978

Additional Notes

Basic course

1   The basic course of immunization against diphtheria, pertussis, tetanus and poliomyelitis should begin at 3 months of age and be completed as early as possible because of the need to protect the young infant against pertussis. The maximum response to all three components of triple (DTPer/Vac/Ads) vaccine will be secured if there is an interval of 6–8 weeks between the first and second dose and 4–6 months between the second and third dose.

The recommended schedule is:

1st dose	*2nd dose*	*3rd dose*
3 months	$4\frac{1}{2}$–5 months	$8\frac{1}{2}$–11 months

If whooping cough is prevalent an alternative course of triple vaccine with one month's interval between the first and second and second and third doses might be considered. However, such a course should be followed at 12–18 months of age by a dose of DT/Vac/Ads vaccine since the intervals of one month are considered not to give adequate basic immunity against diphtheria and tetanus.

If the basic course of vaccination is interrupted the course should be resumed with the appropriate subsequent intervals without repetition of earlier doses. If the basic immunization is commenced after the age of 3 years, pertussis vaccine may be omitted and diphtheria/tetanus toxoid and oral poliovaccine given.

Reinforcing doses
2 Reinforcing doses of diphtheria/tetanus vaccine (DT/Vac/Ads) after the basic course.

There should preferably be an interval of at least 3 years between the last dose of the basic course and the boosting dose of diphtheria/tetanus vaccine which is usually given at school entrance or at entry to nursery school. A booster dose of tetanus vaccine (Tet/Vac/Ads) is recommended on leaving school, entering higher education or on commencing employment unless this has been administered within the past year following injury. Reinforcing doses of poliovaccine are advised on school entry, on leaving school, entering higher education or going to work, and for travel abroad to countries where poliomyelitis is endemic.

Measles vaccine
3 Measles vaccine should be offered to all susceptible children from the second year of life to puberty. It is important to recognize that the following groups are at special risk:
i   children from the age of one year upwards in residential care,
ii   children entering nursery school or other establishment accepting children for day care,
iii children with serious physical incapacity who are likely to develop severe illness as the result of natural measles infection. The use of immunoglobulin with the vaccine should be considered in these cases. Contra-indications to vaccination should be observed especially in immune-deficient states.

BCG vaccine
4 BCG vaccine is given as a routine to children aged 11–13 years who are tuberculin negative irrespective of whether there is a history of BCG vaccination at an earlier age. BCG vaccine should be given at birth to children who come from environments where there is a high risk of contracting tuberculosis e.g. certain immigrant families. Tuberculin-negative contacts of known cases of tuberculosis should be given BCG vaccine. Certain virus infections, such as measles, rubella and chickenpox, can suppress the tuberculin test for about 4–6 weeks. For this reason the tuberculin test should not be carried out in the 6 weeks after rubella or measles vaccinations, nor should BCG vaccine be given within 3 weeks after these vaccinations (see note 7). Girls are normally offered rubella vaccine at about the same time as BCG. One suggested schedule is to carry out tuberculin testing, read the test and give BCG to the negative responders then wait 3 weeks for rubella vaccination. Alternatively, rubella vaccination may be done first and 6 weeks later the tuberculin testing and BCG programme carried out.

Rubella vaccine
5   Rubella vaccine may be given to all girls at the age of 11–13 years irrespective of a history of rubella, which cannot be relied upon as evidence of actual immunity. Vaccination is also strongly recommended for adult women of child bearing age who are seronegative and therefore susceptible. A warning must be given to avoid pregnancy for 8 weeks after inoculation of rubella vaccine in order to avoid the possible risk of harm to the fetus.

Oral poliomyelitis vaccine
6   Unvaccinated parents should receive oral poliovaccine at the same time as the first dose of oral poliovaccine is given to their baby and arrangements should be made for the parents to complete their basic course of immunization. If the baby's mother who has not herself received poliovaccine is within the first 4 months of pregnancy immunization of the baby should be delayed until the fourth month of pregnancy has passed. If the circumstances are such that immunization of the baby should not be delayed i.e. a risk exists of natural infection from an outbreak, both mother and baby should be given oral poliovaccine.
7   An interval of not less than 3 weeks should normally be allowed to lapse between the administration of any two live vaccines, whichever is given first.

2   Immunization of travellers

Travellers to other countries, particularly tropical or underdeveloped countries, require a variety of immunizations, partly for their own protection, partly to prevent the spread of epidemic disease, and in the three diseases of smallpox, yellow fever and cholera, to fulfil legal requirements of entry. Such regulations apply not only to the country of destination, but to all ports-of-call on the journey. Information on the necessary vaccinations is obtained from the annual publications of the World Health Organization and the National Communicable Diseases Centre, Atlanta, Georgia, USA but may be checked if necessary with the consulates of the countries to be visited.

(a) *Typhoid and paratyphoid*
Travellers to underdeveloped countries should be protected against typhoid. TAB vaccine containing tyhpoid and para-typhoid A and B organisms killed by heat and preserved in phenol is traditionally used. TAB is available combined with tetanus toxoid (TABT) or with cholera vaccine (TAB Cho). Severe local and febrile general reactions with TAB are common. A new and more effective monovalent anti-typhoid vaccine may eventually replace TAB vaccine.

(b) *Poliomyelitis*
All travellers should be protected against poliomyelitis.

(c) *Yellow fever*

Yellow fever vaccine contains live attenuated virus prepared on chick embryos and frozen and dried for storage. It is reconstituted in cold normal saline immediately before use, and only one dose of 0·5 ml given subcutaneously is required. An international vaccination certificate is valid for ten years but re-inoculation may be indicated earlier in the face of an epidemic. Protection is necessary only for those travelling through, or living in, infected areas such as tropical Africa or South and Central America, or for laboratory workers handling infected material, and reactions are rare. Vaccination of infants under 1 year of age is not normally advised owing to the occasional risk of encephalitis. This vaccine is given only at special centres, listed in the Notice to Travellers issued by the Department of Health. The vaccine is not given to individuals known to be hypersensitive to egg protein, polymixin or neomycin.

(d) *Cholera*

Vaccines must contain the requisite number of killed *Vibrio cholerae* of the classical biotypes. Field trials have shown that such vaccines provide some protection against infections caused by both the classical and El Tor biotypes. Primary vaccination consists of two subcutaneous injections of 0·5 ml and 1·0 ml preferably separated by an interval of 4–6 weeks. The dose for children is 0·2 ml and 0·4 ml and the vaccine is not advised under one year of age. Painful local reactions are common. Immunity is short-lived, and if exposure to infection continues revaccination should be carried out within 6 months.

(e) *Smallpox*

An international certificate is required for many countries of the world and is valid for 3 years.

(f) *Typhus*

Cox's killed vaccine, stored at 5°C, is only necessary in endemic areas and there is no international certificate. The dose is 2 subcutaneous injections of 1 ml at 1 week's interval, and annual booster doses are necessary. The dose for children is 0·3–0·5 ml.

3 General contra-indications to vaccinations

(a) Vaccinations are postponed if the patient is suffering from an acute febrile illness, other than a 'head cold'.

(b) Live vaccines are not given to pregnant women, particularly in the early months, unless the risk of acquiring disease is substantial.

(c) Live vaccines are not given to patients on corticosteroid or immunosuppressive drugs or receiving X-ray treatment, or to patients suffering from diseases which impair immune reactions, such as leukaemia, Hodgkin's disease or other lymphoma, or from immunity defects such as agammaglobulinaemia.

4. Intervals between immunizing procedures
Although there is only slender evidence on the clashing effects of vaccines given at varying intervals, the following general recommendations may be put forward.

(a) Almost any combination of killed vaccines and a single live vaccine may be given at one time.

(b) An interval of not less than three weeks is desirable between any two live vaccines. If time does not permit, it is better to give live vaccines at the same time, rather than at a shorter interval, as in the latter event, the later vaccines may not be fully effective because of interference. There is no evidence that it is harmful to give live vaccines at the same time, but rather that interference may occur.

5. Further details on immunization and specific contraindications
Further details on diphtheria, tetanus, pertussis, poliomyelitis, measles, BCG, rubella, typhoid, cholera, smallpox, anthrax, influenza and rabies vaccinations and on protective measures in viral hepatitis and malaria will be found in the appropriate chapters.

CHAPTER 3

Viral Infections

Viruses are smaller than other micro-organisms and are not normally visible with a light microscope. Although they may survive and freely transmit disease in the environment, they are capable of multiplication or replication only within the living cells of a host.

All living cells, including bacteria and rickettsiae, contain nucleic acid in both RNA (ribonucleic acid) and DNA (desoxyribonucleic acid) forms. Viruses differ fundamentally, in that they contain either RNA or DNA but not both. This is a useful biochemical basis for a classification of the important human viruses.

Classification of viruses

(A) *RNA Viruses*

1 *Myxovirus*
  Influenza A, B and C

2 *Paramyxovirus*
  Parainfluenza
  Respiratory syncytial
  Measles
  Mumps

3 *Rhabdovirus*
  Rabies

4 *Picornavirus*
  Poliovirus
  Coxsackie
  ECHO
  Rhinovirus

5 *Togavirus*
  Rubella
  Arbovirus (Alpha group–encephalitis
              Flavi group–yellow fever)
  Hepatitis A and B
  Arena virus (Lassa fever, lymphocytic choriomeningitis)

6 *Double stranded*
  Reo, orbi and rotavirus

(C) *Unclassified*
Ebola and Marburg viruses

(B) *DNA Viruses*

1 *Herpesvirus*
  Herpes simplex
  Varicella/zoster
  Cytomegalovirus
  Epstein–Barr virus

2 *Adenovirus*

3 *Papovavirus*

4 *Poxvirus*
  Smallpox
  Vaccinia
  Orf

Immunity in viral infections

Viral infections stimulate the production of globulin antibodies in the serum. IgM type antibodies are produced first but disappear after a few months whereas IgG type antibodies appear a little later and persist in the serum for a long time. These antibodies terminate the viraemic phase and generally protect against future infection. They cannot however enter the host's cells where replication of virus is taking place and probably play no part in the eventual recovery from infection which depends on cell-mediated immune response. Interferon, a protein substance produced by the cells, also helps in the recovery process. IgA antibodies are believed to confer immunity at mucosal surfaces.

Some viruses exist in a number of antigenically distinct strains, and so in spite of antibody production, repeated infections occur throughout life, and this is particularly true of viral respiratory tract infections. Others, such as measles, rubella and mumps, exist only in a single stable strain, so that a single attack of the disease occurs.

In the therapeutic field, preparations of human immunoglobulin are available and contain specific antibody to a number of common viruses. The preparations are able to prevent the occurrence of several common virus diseases, such as measles and virus A hepatitis, when given early in the incubation period at a time when the virus is at the vulnerable extracellular stage. When the disease has developed and the virus is replicating intracellularly, immunoglobulin has little or no effect on the subsequent course of the illness. Interferon is not available for routine treatment as attempts to produce it in quantity have not been successful. Animal sources of interferon are of no value in humans, as the substance is specific to each animal species.

Diagnosis of virus infections

Some viral infections can be diagnosed accurately from the characteristic clinical syndrome, but in many, diagnosis depends on laboratory methods. Direct microscopic examination of specimens is usually of no value, and the main techniques for diagnosis are the isolation of the virus and the demonstration of a rising antibody level. Virus isolation is normally carried out in tissue culture of which monkey kidney, human amnion or the more permanent HeLa cell lines are among the more commonly used. Antibody rise is detected by the examination of paired serum specimens, the first taken as early as possible in the illness and the second about 2 weeks later. Usually, a fourfold rise in antibody titre is taken as satisfactory evidence of an active or very recent infection. Unfortunately, both tissue culture and antibody demonstration are slow methods and so are of limited value in the early diagnosis of infection. However, in recent years, techniques have developed for rapid identification of many virus infections, e.g. electronmicroscopy (herpes simplex, varicella-zoster, variola, vaccinia, orf and rotavirus); radioimmunoassay and passive haemagglutination (hepatitis B); and immunofluorescence (respiratory syncytial virus, rabies, herpes simplex).

Current techniques in virology have led to the development of successful vaccines against poliomyelitis, measles and rubella. At present, viral chemotherapy is in its infancy and no highly successful drug is available. There is still the need for the development of more active and less toxic antiviral drugs, and a parallel need for more rapid methods of laboratory diagnosis for the application of such drugs.

CHAPTER 4

Herpesvirus Infections

Herpesvirus hominis, Epstein–Barr virus, varicella zoster virus and cytomegalovirus are important members of the herpesvirus group. The infections are widespread in the community and tend to be mild or subclinical in nature. The group commonly cause persistent or latent infections resulting in an infective carrier state.

A Herpes simplex infections

Herpes simplex infections caused by the *Herpesvirus hominis* are almost universal in man. Apart from 'cold sores', the commonest clinical manifestation is an acute ulcerative stomatitis. Following infection, many patients become long-term carriers. Burnett has suggested that this is one of the most ancient of human infections, because of the mild clinical illness, the ability to sustain the infection in small closed communities such as primitive tribes and the occurrence of an almost identical virus in other primates.

Epidemiology
Primary infection can occur at any age but is most common in the very young child. Babies in the first few months of life are usually immune because of transferred maternal antibody. Most primary infections are clinically inapparent and can only be detected by a rise in serum antibody. Clinically apparent infections most commonly affect the mouth, conjunctiva, skin or female genital tract. These infections are short-lived and heal completely, but the virus may persist for many years in the cells of the skin, particularly round the mouth and also in the trigeminal ganglion, in spite of protective levels of antibody in the blood. From time to time, because of some systemic upset, there is reactivation of the latent virus with the formation of new lesions. Both the primary and the recurrent lesions are highly infectious. Infection spreads by droplet infection, by close personal contact as in kissing, and by contaminated utensils. Infection is more common, and occurs at an earlier age, in overcrowded or unhygienic social conditions. Two types of the virus are recognized. Type 1 is the cause of most oral, conjunctival and cutaneous infections and Type 2 is the cause of most genital infection.

A closely related virus, *Herpesvirus simiae* (formerly herpes B virus), is commonly found in monkeys. When man is infected, usually as a result of a monkey bite, a highly fatal encephalitis may result.

Incubation period
This is usually 4–5 days.

Clinical picture
Herpetic ulcerative stomatitis
This is the most common clinical manifestation and it occurs particularly in young children. The onset is abrupt with fever,

general malaise, irritability and soreness of the mouth. A rash then appears on the skin around the lips, or occasionally more widely on the face and neck. The rash consists of painful vesicles set on an inflamed base and these may be single or in groups of varying size. In a few cases there is also a generalized discrete vesicular rash on the trunk and limbs. At the same time, wide-spread painful ulceration develops in the mouth affecting the tongue, gums, palate and buccal mucosa. The mouth lesions are shallow inflamed ulcers, covered with whitish exudate, which bleed when touched. There is excess blood-tinged saliva in the mouth, which causes dribbling in young children. The skin vesicles and mouth ulceration persist for a week or longer, together with sustained fever; the local lymph glands become enlarged. Young children frequently refuse to eat or drink.

After healing, the mucosal lesions do not recur, but the skin lesions may re-appear over a period of many years, either as single or grouped vesicles, usually termed 'cold sores'. The common precipitating cause of a recurrence is a febrile illness, but it may follow trauma, fatigue or exposure to cold or sunlight.

Less common clinical presentations

1   *Generalized infection of the newborn.* This is a rare but frequently fatal form, presenting a few days after birth, with vomiting, convulsions, skin lesions, hepatosplenomegaly and circulatory collapse. Most of these cases are caused by Type 2 virus acquired from the mother suffering from genital herpes.

2   *Keratoconjunctivitis.* This primary form of infection presents with painful conjunctivitis, usually unilateral. This infection may be recurrent with the formation of dendritic ulcers leading to chronic scarring and damage to vision.

3   *Genital herpes.* This primary infection presents with vesicular or ulcerative lesions on the vulva and cervix in the female and on the penis in the male and are commonly recurrent. These conditions are being increasingly recognized at VD clinics and in adults are almost certainly sexually transmitted.

4   *Herpetic whitlow.* This is probably a true viral wound infection and presents as an indolent inflammatory lesion arising at the site of a minor skin trauma, usually on a finger. Superficial vesiculation is often present at some stage. If the

diagnosis is suspected, surgical incision is to be avoided as the lesion is self-limiting.

5   *Eczema herpeticum.* In patients suffering from chronic eczema, primary herpes infection of the skin causes a serious illness. In the eczematous areas, confluent vesiculation occurs, which breaks down leaving raw and weeping areas. There is high fever with a severe systemic upset and the illness may be fatal. The older name for this condition was Kaposi's varicelliform eruption, but this also embraced a similar condition caused by the vaccinia virus.

6   *Herpes encephalitis.* Rarely, the herpes virus may invade the nervous system, either during primary infection or during a recurrence. Herpes encephalitis is a serious illness, presenting with meningeal irritation, cranial nerve lesions, convulsions, and impaired consciousness leading to coma. Local areas of oedema and necrosis may lead to localizing neurological signs, sometimes suggestive of a space-occupying lesion. The mortality is higher than in most other forms of encephalitis, varying from 20 to 60 per cent in different series and the survivors often show evidence of permanent brain damage. This condition is different from the more usual post-infectious type of encephalitis, which complicates viral diseases, in that the virus directly invades the brain and can be isolated from biopsy specimens and occasionally from the CSF.

Diagnosis

The diagnosis of herpes simplex infection can be readily confirmed by the isolation of the virus from superficial lesions and by rising serum antibody levels. In encephalitis, a brain biopsy is necessary to establish the diagnosis rapidly. The virus may be detected by electron microscopy or immunofluorescent microscopy and grows quickly in tissue cultures, so that confirmation is possible within a very few days. Acute ulcerative stomatitis in a child is practically always due to herpesvirus. Recurrent aphthous ulceration of the mouth in adults is not due to herpesvirus.

Prognosis

Generalized infection of the newborn, and herpes encephalitis, although rare, are both commonly fatal. Eczema herpeticum is occasionally fatal. Keratoconjunctivitis may permanently impair vision. The other more common forms of infection are benign.

Treatment
This is largely supportive, and aims at the relief of symptoms with analgesics and mouth washes, and the maintenance of fluid intake. Antibiotics are often prescribed but have no effect on the course of the illness.

The antiviral drugs idoxuridine (IDU), cytosine arabinoside (cytarabine) and adenine arabinoside (vidarabine) are active *in vitro* against herpesvirus. In skin infections, local applications of idoxuridine may shorten the duration of the lesions and reduce the infectivity. In conjunctival infections, local trifluorothymidine is increasingly used in preference to other antiviral drugs. In encephalitis IDU has been abandoned as being ineffective and hazardous. Adenine arabinoside (vidarabine) is the preferred drug and is being used although there is little evidence, as yet, that it is beneficial. These drugs are cytotoxic and are liable to produce troublesome side effects, particularly depression of the bone marrow and damage to the gastrointestinal mucosa.

B Cytomegalovirus infection

Intrauterine infection of the fetus is fairly common and is increasingly recognized. This may result in severe generalized disease in the neonate with jaundice, hepatosplenomegaly and thrombocytopenia, but more often results in brain damage alone. It is estimated that more than 400 children born in England each year suffer gross mental retardation from this cause and many more suffer a lesser degree of mental impairment.

In adults and older children, subclinical infection occurs very commonly as shown by antibody surveys. Clinical illness may occur and the following overlapping syndromes have been described:
(a) Pyrexial illness without localizing features.
(b) Hepatitis, often with prolonged pyrexia.
(c) Glandular fever-like illness with negative Paul–Bunnell, sometimes accompanied by thrombocytopenia.
(d) Acute polyneuritis of the Guillain–Barre type.
(e) Post-perfusion syndrome—this is a severe glandular fever-

like illness which may follow the administration of fresh blood in open heart surgery. This is a serious condition which may end fatally.

(f) Following organ transplant surgery, there may be a pyrexial reactivation of infection with this virus, with severe pneumonitis. This is another serious condition which may be fatal.

The diagnosis is confirmed by the isolation of the virus in tissue culture from urine, blood or saliva and by the demonstration of high antibody levels in the blood.

Experimental studies in the production and use of a vaccine are now beginning but there are no other effective treatments of preventive measures.

CHAPTER 5

Glandular Fever

Glandular fever (infectious mononucleosis) is a benign infectious disease with a variable clinical picture, in which fever, lymphadenopathy and sore throat are common features. The diagnosis is confirmed by the recognition of atypical monocytes in the peripheral blood and a positive Paul–Bunnell reaction. The Epstein–Barr virus is the cause of the condition.

Epidemiology

The disease was first described in 1889, and its association with atypical mononuclear cells in the blood was established in 1920. The causative agent is thought to be the Epstein–Barr virus (EB virus) which belongs to the herpesvirus group, and rising antibody titres to this virus are found in most Paul–Bunnell positive cases. The Paul–Bunnell or the alternative Monospot test and the presence of atypical mononuclear cells are still the mainstay of clinical diagnosis because of their speed and simplicity, EB virus antibody tests being used more in research studies.

The disease occurs in most parts of the world and is well recognized in all developed countries. Cases are usually sporadic, but prolonged localized epidemics occur, mostly in schools and institutions. The annual incidence of clinical cases in Britain may be as high as 1 case per 2000 of the population. The disease probably spreads by droplet infection, and kissing has been incriminated as a mode of spread. Infectivity is not high and its duration is unknown. All ages are susceptible, but the disease is more common, at least in its more severe forms, among young adults. Second attacks have been recorded. Surveys among contacts have shown that mild and atypical cases occur and that healthy contacts may show evidence of infection. EB virus antibody surveys show that 30 per cent of children have been infected by the age of 5 years, and a much higher percentage in young adults, so that mild or inapparent clinical infections must be very common from an early age.

Incubation period
The incubation period is usually 10–15 days, but may be much longer on occasions.

Clinical picture
The onset is often insidious with tiredness, vague malaise and headache being present for a week or longer before the disease is established. Occasionally the disease presents abruptly with high fever.

Fever is usually present, but is variable in degree and duration, lasting from 2 or 3 days to 2 or 3 weeks.

Lymphadenopathy is usually present at some stage in the illness. The neck glands are usually involved and may be visibly enlarged. The axillary glands are also quite commonly involved. The enlarged glands are discrete and slightly tender. The spleen is palpably enlarged in about half the cases.

In most cases of glandular fever, sore throat occurs at some stage of the illness, but in some cases this becomes the predominant feature, interfering with swallowing and with speech. Inspection of the throat, in these cases, shows extensive exudate on the tonsils, with gross inflammation and oedema of the fauces, which completely distorts the normal anatomy. Rarely the inflammation may cause airway obstruction sufficiently severe to require tracheotomy. This condition which is termed anginose glandular fever, is now the commonest cause of severe throat infection in this country. The sore throat, with or without exudate, may persist for several days or for a week or more.

A crescent of pinpoint petechiae may occur at the junction of the hard and soft palates, particularly in the anginose cases. Occasionally linear or circular papules occur at the same site.

Swelling of the lachrymal gland with oedema of the upper eyelid is an occasional minor feature.

In a small minority of cases a rash appears at some stage of the illness; this is most common in young adults, and usually takes the form of a coarse generalized maculopapular erythema. In patients treated with ampicillin the incidence of severe papular rash is much higher, although there is no lasting hypersensitivity to ampicillin in these patients.

Jaundice is another uncommon manifestation of the illness, and shows features similar to viral hepatitis, but is generally mild and short-lived. A larger percentage of cases have a raised serum aminotransferase (SALT) level, and this is taken as evidence of a subclinical hepatitis.

The disease continues for 2 or 3 weeks, with any combination of these features, and then gradually subsides. In some cases, notably in adolescence, there is persistent malaise, fatigue and sweating for 2–3 months after the acute febrile illness has settled. In many of these cases, the spleen remains enlarged and the Paul–Bunnell test remains positive.

Complications

A number of rare complications have been described, including:
1   A haemorrhagic tendency leading to epistaxis, gastrointestinal haemorrhage or ruptured spleen.
2   Haemolytic anaemia.
3   Thrombocytopenic purpura.
4   Myocarditis.
5   Pericarditis.
6   Lymphocytic meningitis.
7   Polyneuritis.
8   Encephalitis.

Diagnosis

The symptoms, lymphadenopathy, and the characteristic throat appearances, often lead to a clinical diagnosis.

On occasions, glandular fever must be distinguished from conditions as varied as rubella, measles, secondary syphilis, drug reactions, lymphadenoma, leukaemia, agranulocytosis, tonsillitis, quinsy, diphtheria, mumps, viral hepatitis, leptospirosis, viral meningitis and acute neurological disease.

Two rare but increasingly recognized conditions which mimic glandular fever closely are the adult forms of toxoplasmosis and cytomegalovirus infection.

Laboratory diagnosis depends on examination of peripheral blood films and the Paul–Bunnell reaction. The blood film shows atypical mononuclear cells, which usually represent 10–25 per cent of the differential count; this may be associated with a lymphocytosis, or a neutrophil leucocytosis or, indeed, a leucopenia. The Paul–Bunnell reaction detects the presence of heterophil antibodies capable of agglutinating sensitized sheep red cell suspensions. In true cases of glandular fever, this antibody is present to a titre of 1/64 or more and is adsorbed by ox red cells, but not by guinea-pig kidney cells, while the reverse is true in certain serum sensitizations. The Monospot test is a useful screening test, being a faster but slightly less sensitive version of the Paul–Bunnell test. The Paul–Bunnell reaction may be positive as early as the end of the 1st week but it may be considerably delayed even as late as the 4th week of illness. The reaction may remain positive for several months.

In a minority of cases, otherwise typical of glandular fever, the Paul–Bunnell reaction remains negative, and this happens particularly in milder cases and in young children. Rising EB virus antibody titres are found in positive Paul–Bunnell cases, and occasionally in negative cases. Isolation of the EB virus is technically difficult and is not performed routinely.

Prognosis

Practically all cases eventually make a full recovery. Death only occurs very rarely, followed a ruptured spleen or respiratory obstruction.

Treatment

Most cases remain at home, with symptomatic treatment and bed rest during the febrile stage. Antibiotics have no place in treatment even in the anginose form of the disease, and ampicillin is particularly to be avoided. There is growing evidence that a short course of prednisolone is of value in the anginose case. The inflammatory swelling is reduced (sometimes quite dramatically) and as a result the patient feels better. Rare complicated cases may require more active treatment, such as the surgical removal of a ruptured spleen, tracheotomy for airway obstruction or artificial respiration for polyneuritis.

Prevention
Nothing can be done to prevent the spread of this disease in the community and quarantine of contacts is unnecessary. Cases are isolated as far as possible until recovery.

CHAPTER 6

Chickenpox and Herpes Zoster

A Chickenpox

Chickenpox is a mild, highly infectious virus disease, with a rash of central distribution.

Epidemiology
The causative agent of chickenpox is the varicella-zoster virus (V-Z virus) which belongs to the herpesvirus group. The virus is not easily cultured but may be isolated from the nasopharynx and fresh vesicular skin lesions, although not from lesions which have reached the crusting stage. Infectivity is greater when mucosal lesions are present; it is at a peak from the onset of symptoms until cropping of the rash has stopped (about 5 days), and continues until the skin lesions become dry and crusted. Transmission of infection is usually by droplet infection, but may be by direct skin contact or by recently contaminated articles. The disease occurs throughout the world, and is endemic in all large cities. There is no seasonal prevalence, and local epidemics occur at irregular intervals. The disease occurs mainly in childhood; it is uncommon in adults, in whom the

B*

attack tends to be more severe. One attack confers permanent immunity so that second attacks are rare.

Incubation period
This is usually 13–17 days, with limits of 10–21 days.

Clinical picture
In children, the appearance of the rash is often the first sign of illness, although in severe cases and particularly in adults there may be a prodromal period lasting up to 2–3 days, in which pyrexia, headache, vomiting and malaise occur. A sore throat commonly results from mucosal lesions.

A macular rash first appears on the trunk, and soon afterwards on the head and limbs. Fresh crops of macules may continue to appear for the first three days of the rash. The macules change in a few hours to papules surmounted by a superficial clear vesicle. The vesicles vary in size, are often oval in shape and are unilocular. The clear vesicles quickly change to opaque pustules, which soon rupture or dry to form crusts. The process of maturation from macules to crusts takes from 1–3 days, but many lesions abort at an early stage. The crusts separate in about a week, and only an unusually large or deep individual lesion leaves a permanent scar. The rapid maturation of the lesions, and the occurrence of cropping, soon results in the appearance of lesions at all stages from macules to crusts at one time. The rash is central in distribution, and so is most dense on the trunk and head, is less dense on the upper arms and thighs and is least dense on the forearms and lower legs. It tends to be more profuse in protected areas such as the axillae, and on flexor surfaces.

The rash may be sparse or profuse, and its density determines the severity of the fever and systemic upset. Adults tend to have a profuse rash and a severe systemic upset. Itching is a variable feature. Lesions commonly occur on the buccal mucosa, palate or tongue, the lesions appearing as circular yellow ulcers with an inflamed areola.

Complications
1 Post-infectious encephalitis occurs rarely. It usually takes the form of a pure cerebellar disturbance with gross ataxia, incoordination and intention tremor. This form has a uniformly

good prognosis. Rarely the complication takes the more severe form of a meningoencephalomyelitis similar to the variety which follows measles.

2 Pneumonitis may complicate severe attacks of the disease, particularly in adults. Symptoms include dyspnoea and cyanosis with a dry cough. Chest X-ray shows nodular opacities scattered densely throughout the lung fields. Some nodules persist and slowly calcify after recovery, leaving a permanent scattering of small calcified opacities on chest X-ray.

Patients on long-term corticosteroid or immunosuppressive therapy, particularly for a disease such as leukaemia, which causes further immune compromise, may suffer from virulent or fatal chickenpox. The illness is prolonged, the rash is dense even semi-confluent with deep ulcerating lesions and a complicating pneumonitis is common.

Diagnosis

At one time smallpox was the most important condition to be differentiated from chickenpox and even now, until the eradication of smallpox is complete, this should be considered in any patient returning from abroad with atypical chickenpox. Vaccination history; prodromal illness; evolution, distribution and morphology of the rash will generally allow a definite diagnosis, but if doubt remains, laboratory investigations would be carried out. Other causes of a generalized papulovesicular rash include eczema herpeticum, eczema vaccinatum, drug eruption, pustular impetigo, Stevens–Johnson syndrome, insect bites and certain Coxsackie virus infections.

Prognosis

Usually the illness is benign. Rarely death occurs, either in immune compromised children or from encephalitis or pneumonitis.

Treatment

In uncomplicated cases little is required in the way of treatment. Bed rest is only necessary while fever persists; calamine cream may be used if the rash is irritating. In encephalitis, only supportive measures are necessary.

In pneumonitis, oxygen is necessary as cyanosis is frequently present. Broad spectrum antibiotics, corticosteroids and anti-viral chemotherapy in the form of cytosine arabinoside or adenine arabinoside are frequently given although the value of all these measures remains doubtful. Virulent chickenpox in the immune compromised patient is treated similarly with in addition a large dose of hyperimmune zoster immunoglobulin (ZIG), but again the value of the therapy is very doubtful.

Prevention
Cases are kept indoors for a week, or until the lesions are crusted and dry. Isolation within the home and quarantine of school contacts are ineffectual and unnecessary measures.

Patients on corticosteroid or immunosuppressive therapy must be specially warned about chickenpox. If such a patient becomes a contact, particularly within the family, a dose of zoster immunoglobulin will prevent or modify the disease if given early in the incubation period.

B   Herpes zoster

Herpes zoster or 'shingles' is also caused by the V-Z virus. Following an attack of chickenpox, the V-Z virus may persist permanently in the sensory nerves and root ganglia. If immunity to chickenpox has sufficiently declined, reactivation of this latent infection may occur and an eruption appears in the skin area supplied by the nerve. The eruption is infectious and chickenpox commonly occurs in susceptible contacts. In the reverse situation, there is little evidence that herpes zoster occurs as a result of contact with chickenpox. Zoster is most common in middle-aged or elderly people. The incidence of zoster is higher among patients with underlying disease in which immunity mechanisms are impaired such as leukaemia and Hodgkin's disease. Occasionally zoster is recurrent.

Clinical picture
The condition presents with pain and paraesthesia along the course of a sensory nerve for several days before the appearance of the eruption, which consists of plaques of vesicles set in an inflammatory base. The eruption is confined to the segmental distribution of one or more spinal nerves, or the sensory division of a cranial nerve; it is unilateral and does not extend

across the mid-line of the body. The vesicles break down to form moist weeping crusts within about a week and the crusts dry and separate over a further period of 1–2 weeks leaving depigmented anaesthetic areas which may be permanent. Pain and paraesthesia may persist for months after healing.

The commonest sites of infection are the intercostal nerves and the ophthalmic branch of the 5th cranial nerve. Ophthalmic zoster causes a unilateral eruption on the forehead with a severe conjunctivitis which may damage the cornea and impair vision. Zoster of the maxillary branch of the 5th nerve causes a unilateral eruption on the cheek and on the same half of the palate. Zoster of the geniculate ganglion causes a painful eruption of the external auditory meatus often with unilateral facial paralysis (Ramsay–Hunt syndrome).

Complications
1   Meningoencephalitis—a lymphocytic reaction in the CSF occurs commonly in otherwise uncomplicated cases, but in a few patients there may be frank signs of meningeal irritation. Rarely an encephalitis or myelitis may occur.
2   Paralysis of related muscles is another occasional neurological complication.
3   Disseminated zoster—a few chickenpox-like lesions occur commonly away from the zoster area. Very occasionally this rash may be very profuse, particularly in patients with lymphoreticular malignancy or with defective immunity from other causes. In these immune compromised patients there is a considerable mortality.
4   Post-herpetic neuralgia—in occasional patients, usually over 55 years of age, the neuralgic pain may persist severely for months or even years after resolution of the skin lesions. The worst neuralgia tends to follow in patients with extensive skin lesions and residual scarring.

Treatment
Local treatment with 40 per cent idoxuridine in dimethylsulphoxide is of proven benefit, if applied very soon after the appearance of the rash. The area involved is covered in gauze which is kept constantly soaked with the solution for 4 days. By shortening the duration and reducing the severity of the cutaneous lesions, this may prevent the later development of

scarring and post-herpetic neuralgia. This treatment is very expensive; a cheaper five per cent preparation is marketed commercially (Herpid) but is probably of more limited value. If the eye is involved, local atropine is applied to dilate the pupil and prevent adhesions and local antibiotics are applied to prevent secondary infection. Established post-herpetic neuralgia is difficult to treat. If analgesics such as Pentazocine (50–100 mg four-hourly), cool spray and local vibrator massage fail to relieve the condition, then electric percutaneous nerve stimulation may be beneficial.

CHAPTER 7

Smallpox

Smallpox is a serious viral infection, characterized by a pustular rash which is most dense towards the extremities, with a severe systemic upset.

Epidemiology
The causative virus belongs to the pox virus group and exists in two fixed types of greatly differing virulence. The more virulent type causes variola major with a mortality of 40 per cent and the less virulent causes variola minor or alastrim with a mortality of less than 1 per cent.

In the 19th century variola major was endemic throughout the world, but during the last 30 years has become confined to the Indian subcontinent and Indonesia. Importations from the Indian subcontinent occurred sporadically in Britain until recent years. The World Health Organization has carried out its greatest and most successful eradication programme on smallpox and it is now believed that variola major is extinct as a natural disease as no case has been reported from the last endemic foci in India, Pakistan and Bangladesh for two years.

Variola minor was formerly widely endemic in Africa and South America and twice became established in Lancashire during the present century. The WHO programme is continuing against this disease which was confined to a single shrinking focus in Ethiopia and Somalia, which is probably now eradicated.

The last cases of smallpox in Britain occurred in 1973 and in 1978 and these arose from laboratory accidents: as a result new and strict regulations in the handling of dangerous pathogens were introduced.

Cases of smallpox are infectious from the onset of symptoms until the separation of the last crust. The virus can survive in crusts, dust and clothing for several months and infection may arise from these sources. All age groups are susceptible. An attack of the disease confers permanent immunity. Vaccination protects against both types of disease.

Incubation period

This is usually 11–12 days with limits of 7–16 days in variola major and 7–21 days in variola minor.

Clinical picture

In view of the eradication of variola major and the probable eradication of variola minor, only a brief clinical description need be given.

The illness presents with 3–4 days of prodromal symptoms including fever, headache, backache and malaise. The rash first appears on the face and forearms as macules and papules which change after 2–3 days to deep-set vesicles. These mature in a further 2–3 days to pearly pustules which last for several days before drying and breaking down to crusts which separate during the following 1–2 weeks. The rash is most dense on the face, forearms and lower legs and is least dense on the trunk. There is a severe febrile systemic upset and complications include corneal ulceration, bronchopneumonia and myocarditis.

Fulminating, haemorrhagic or confluent varieties occurred in variola major and these were usually fatal, while a mild modified illness could occur in a previously vaccinated person.

Diagnosis

Smallpox must still be considered when a patient arrives from an endemic or a recently cleared area, and is found to have fever and a suspicious rash. Such a patient is isolated and kept under observation until laboratory investigations are carried out.

Chickenpox and generalized vaccinia are the conditions most likely to be confused with smallpox.

Laboratory diagnosis
Specimens are collected and transported in special kits and are only examined in laboratories designated by the Department of Health.

The following specimens are collected:
(a) Scrapings from the base of papules, vesicles or pustules spread on glass slides.
(b) Fluid from vesicles or pustules aspirated into a tuberculin syringe.
(c) Crusts collected in a dry container.
(d) In very early or very late cases blood is collected.

The following investigations are carried out:
(a) Electron microscopy—will reliably show the presence of pox virus but will not distinguish from vaccinia.
(b) Antigen detection by gel diffusion (does not distinguish smallpox from vaccinia).
(c) Culture of virus in fertile hens' eggs is the most sensitive and reliable test, giving results in three days. This will distinguish smallpox from vaccinia or herpes virus infections and can even be used to distinguish variola major and minor.
(d) Blood specimens may be used for virus culture (very early case) or for detecting antibody rises (paired sera).

Treatment and prevention
There is no specific treatment for smallpox. Cases are isolated in a designated smallpox hospital. It has been recommended that these special hospitals remain available for five years after the apparent eradication of smallpox.

Vaccination
This has been the main weapon in the WHO eradication programme. However, routine vaccination of children is no longer necessary in this country. Health Service staff who would have to deal with a suspected case of smallpox require vaccination every three years. It is still common for routine vaccination

to be recommended for many other grades of health workers, but it is increasingly questionable whether this is necessary.

Travellers to, from or through infected smallpox zones require vaccination and the possession of an International Certificate of Vaccination, valid for 3 years. However, about a dozen countries in the world still demand vaccination and certification, several of these countries now having only a remote historical connection with the disease. These requirements now need critical review so that unnecessary smallpox vaccination is reduced.

Although it now appears unlikely that a case of smallpox will occur again in Britain, the control measures which would be used are described, as with modification, similar measures would apply in any other serious imported infection. When a case of smallpox is suspected, the Medical Officer for Environmental Health (MOEH) is immediately informed by telephone and is responsible for preventive measures. A panel of smallpox consultants, appointed by the Department of Health, is available to the MOEH for advice on the diagnosis. The MOEH informs the Department of Health of suspected cases, and information is passed to all general practitioners, hospitals and health authorities. Close contacts are vaccinated within 24 hours, with fresh vaccine, using two insertions and are revaccinated in three days time if there is no evidence of the earlier vaccination 'taking'. Less close contacts are traced and vaccinated on the expanding ring principle. Vaccination is only likely to be successful and to provide protection when carried out within three days of exposure. Antivaccinial immunoglobulin prepared from the blood of recently vaccinated donors provides some passive protection against small pox, when giving during the first half of the incubation period. It is given in a dose of 1500 mg to all first line contacts at the same time as vaccination, unless the contact has a satisfactory previous history of vaccination. Recently methisazone (Marboran) has been used in prophylaxis among contacts. The first trial of this drug in India showed a greater than tenfold reduction in the case rate and mortality. However, more critical trials have since given less promising results. The drug frequently causes vomiting, but it is worth giving to close contacts of variola major, in a dose of 3 g, repeated in 12 hours, in addition to vaccination and immunoglobulin.

Close contacts are kept under daily observation for 16 days in cases of variola major, and for 21 days in variola minor. They are quarantined from work or school for 21 days. Cases are admitted to a hospital reserved for smallpox. The clothing, effects and homes of cases are disinfected. Cases remain in hospital until they are no longer infectious and all possessions are disinfected before the patient is discharged. Ambulances conveying cases to hospital are disinfected and special disinfection is necessary for the disposal of the body of a fatal case. Recommended disinfectants are 1:40 White Fluid and formaldehyde vapour. Special precautions are taken at laboratories handling suspected smallpox material.

On the arrival in this country of a plane or ship carrying a smallpox case, the patient is removed to a smallpox hospital and disinfection is carried out. All travellers and crew are examined and vaccinated. The appropriate Medical Officer for Environmental Health is informed of the destination of each traveller, and observation is maintained throughout the incubation period.

Smallpox is one of the four infectious diseases subject to international control by the World Health Organization.

CHAPTER 8

Vaccinia

For two centuries the prevention of smallpox has depended on vaccination. The vaccinia virus is a hybrid of the pox virus group, antigenically related to the viruses of cowpox and smallpox but not identical with either. After cutaneous infection with vaccinia virus, the individual develops effective immunity against smallpox. Vaccinia lymph is harvested from lesions produced on the skin of living animals, particularly sheep, and is subsequently treated with glycerol and phenol. The lymph is supplied in liquid form, stained with brilliant green, in plastic tubing. When stored in a deep-freeze at minus 10–18°C, it remains potent for twelve months, but only remains potent for one week when left in domestic refrigeration below 10°C. A freeze-dried vaccine, which retains its potency without refrigeration for six months in a temperature climate, is available as a reserve in this country and for use in tropical areas.

The site of election for vaccination is at the junction of the upper and middle thirds of the humerus behind the midline. The skin is cleaned with soap and water and wiped dry. The recommended technique is by 'multiple pressure' in which a drop of vaccine is placed on the skin and a needle held parallel to the skin is pressed through the lymph so that the superficial layer of the skin is disrupted without drawing blood. Some 20 pressures with the needle are used. Alternatively a single superficial quarter-inch scratch is made through the lymph. (In smallpox contacts, two insertions one inch apart are advised, using either method.)

After primary vaccination, an itching papule develops in 3–4 days which matures through a vesicular stage to form a pustule, maximal at the 9th–10th day. The pustule dries to a crust which separates about the 21st day, leaving a permanent scar. Antibody begins to appear in the blood about the 12th day. After revaccination, the pustule develops more rapidly and may remain very small; it is often maximal before the 7th day and antibody also rises more rapidly.

The site of vaccination is inspected on the 7th day and the vaccination is considered successful if a 'major reaction' occurs. A 'major reaction' after primary vaccination is a typical flat Jennerian vesicle (approximately 1-cm diameter).

A 'major reaction' after revaccination is (a) a vesicle or pustule or (b) an area of palpable induration or congestion surrounding a central lesion which may be an ulcer or a scab. Any other reaction is termed an 'equivocal reaction' and the complete absence of a local reaction is recorded as 'no local reaction'. If a 'major reaction' is not obtained, vaccination is repeated with fresh vaccine.

Recent exposure to other infections, systemic illness, failure to thrive, septic conditions, past or present eczema, pregnancy, hypogammaglobulinaemia, leukaemia, lymphoma or other reticuloendothelial malignancy, corticosteroid or immunosuppressive drug therapy are all contra-indications to elective vaccination.

Vaccinia virus may spread from person to person by close

contact, so there is a considerable risk in vaccinating a member of a household in which there is a patient with eczema.

There are no absolute contraindications to the vaccination of close contacts of a case of smallpox. Contacts with eczema, hypogammaglobulinaemia or other contraindication are vaccinated and simultaneously given human antivaccinial immunoglobulin (500–2000 mg) in the other arm.

Complications of vaccination

1 Local sepsis due to secondary bacterial infection occurs occasionally, but is not serious and responds to local or systemic antibiotics.

2 Extraneous lesions due to autoinoculation occur occasionally, and heal at the same time as the primary lesion. These are harmless unless the eye is involved. This complication can be avoided if the infectious nature of the lesion and its hygienic handling are explained to the patient.

3 Allergic erythematous rashes occur occasionally, but are not serious.

4 Generalized vaccinia is an uncommon complication (1 per 20000 primary vaccinations) due to bloodstream spread of the virus. Multiple cutaneous vaccinial lesions develop at the height of the primary lesion with fever and a severe systemic upset. The lesions heal as immunity develops. This condition is more serious if there is a demonstrable immunoglobulin deficiency or an underlying blood dyscrasia. The mortality is low in previously healthy persons.

5 Eczema vaccinatum is an uncommon complication due to the rapid spread of the virus in areas of skin affected by chronic eczema. Groups of vesicles, which may become confluent, appear on the eczematous areas, followed by moist weeping desquamation. There is a severe febrile systemic upset. The mortality is about 10 per cent.

6 Chronic progressive vaccinia (vaccinia gangrenosa or necrosum) is a rare but serious complication due to a failure in the development of immunity, sometimes associated with immunoglobulin deficiency. The primary lesion gradually enlarges and satellite lesions appear, with the slow and widespread development of other lesions in the skin and viscera. This condition is often fatal.

7 Encephalomyelitis is a very rare complication (1 per 100000

primary vaccinations); it is a similar condition to that which may follow other virus infections such as measles. It is more likely to occur after primary vaccination and the symptoms appear about the 10th day. Coma, repeated convulsions and spasticity are common features, the mortality is about 30 per cent and both mental and neurological sequelae occur in some of the survivors.

Treatment
The treatment of the more serious complications is not satisfactory. In generalized vaccinia, chronic progressive vaccinia and eczema vaccinatum, human anti-vaccinial immunoglobulin in repeated doses of 2 g is recommended, but the results are not very encouraging. Methisazone has also been recommended, but is similarly of doubtful value. The treatment of encephalomyelitis is, basically, the management of the unconscious patient; anticonvulsants are necessary but corticosteroids are of doubtful value.

CHAPTER 9

Measles

Measles is an acute viral infectious disease commencing with fever and upper respiratory catarrh. Koplik's spots appear in the mouth during the first few days, and are followed by a generalized maculopapular rash.

Epidemiology
The causative virus belongs to the paramyxovirus group and is closely related to the viruses of rinderpest and canine distemper. The virus may be isolated by tissue culture, but it does not survive for long periods outside the human body.

The disease occurs throughout the world. In secluded communities, where it has been absent for a generation, severe epidemics with a high mortality may occur. In underdeveloped malnourished communities such as in West Africa, measles has a mortality of more than 10 per cent. In developed countries such as Britain, measles is a mild disease with a mortality of about 2 deaths per 10000 notified cases. There has been a steady fall in mortality since the beginning of the century. This fall has accelerated in the past 35 years, since antibiotics have been available. More recently, the mortality has again fallen with the introduction of community vaccination.

Measles is rare in the first 6 months of life, because of transferred passive immunity from the mother. This immunity gradually wanes, but attacks in children of 6–9 months of age are less common and tend to be mild. The greatest incidence is in the 1–7 years age group, and respiratory complications are commoner in the first half of this group.

Measles causes immunosuppression which may predispose to secondary infection and the risk of respiratory complications is increased by poor nutrition, overcrowded homes and poor standards of general care. Physically or mentally handicapped children are particularly at risk. Children in good social conditions tend to contract measles during school age. The great majority of people have had an attack of measles before the end of childhood.

The disease is highly infectious, from a day or two before the onset of symptoms until about five days after the appearance of the rash. The source of infection is always from an existing case, and spread is by droplet infection. One attack usually confers permanent immunity, so that second attacks are very rare.

In Britain epidemics of measles used to occur every second year, each lasting for about six months. Since the introduction of routine vaccination against measles, the previous epidemic peaks are less marked, although the disease continues unchanged in the unvaccinated half of the child population.

Incubation period
This is usually 10–11 days, with limits of 7–21 days.

Clinical picture
The onset is abrupt with fever and diffuse upper respiratory catarrh. This prodromal period lasts about four days with continual pyrexia but occasionally may be extended to seven days. The child is miserable, lethargic, refuses food and may vomit. The

eyes become pink and watery, there is nasal discharge and sneezing, and a troublesome dry cough. In more than 90 per cent of cases, Koplik's spots appear on the 2nd or 3rd day. They are tiny, off-white granules, set on a small red macule, and are most often seen on the buccal mucosa, opposite the molar teeth. They are usually sparse.

Less common features of the prodromal period are:

1   laryngeal involvement with hoarseness and laryngeal stridor;
2   gastrointestinal involvement with persistent vomiting and diarrhoea;
3   fleeting prodromal rashes, which may be urticarial or erythematous.

The true rash of measles appears on the neck, on about the 4th day of the illness, and spreads, within 2–3 days, firstly to the face and trunk, and then to the limbs. The early lesions are discrete macules, these soon develop into larger maculopapules, which become irregularly confluent. Confluent areas of rash are often found over pressure areas. The fever and respiratory catarrh persist throughout the period of the rash, although the Koplik's spots soon degenerate into red roughened areas.

The facial rash, conjunctivitis and respiratory catarrh give the child a highly typical bloated and bleary appearance. The rash persists for 2–4 days before fading, and often leaves characteristic staining, which persists for a further few days. The staining is due to leakage of blood cells into the area of the rash, and varies in colour from deep purple to light brown, and does not fade on pressure. Rarely, fine desquamation may follow the rash. As the rash fades, the temperature returns to normal, the catarrh clears, and in a very few days the child is active, lively and hungry, although the cough may persist into convalescence.

Types of measles

(a) Modified measles—a very mild attenuated attack of measles with a prolonged incubation period may follow partial protection with passive immunity or in young infants with residual maternal antibodies. The rash is scanty and evolves rapidly and Koplik's spots may be absent.

(b) Measles in the tropics—in malnourished tropical communities measles often produces a severe protracted illness with skin desquamation and abscess formation, persistent diarrhoea and bronchopneumonia. The mortality is high.

(c) Atypical measles—children who have previously received killed-virus measles vaccine may develop severe atypical disease if they later contract the infection. Killed-virus vaccines are no longer in use.

(d) Measles in the immunosuppressed—in leukaemic children on immunosuppressant therapy or in cases of congenital immune deficiency measles may be a severe or fatal illness. The rash may be sparse or even non-existent and the children suffer from protracted giant-cell pneumonitis.

Complications
A recent MRC survey of the complications of measles showed four per cent of cases developed bronchitis or pneumonia, 2·5 per cent an otitis media and 0·4 per cent a neurological complication.

1   Respiratory tract
Secondary bacterial infection appears to play a large part in the development of respiratory complications. They occur most commonly in children aged 10 months to 3 years, and particularly those living in poor social conditions.

(*a*) *Otitis media.* This is recognized by redness, and later, bulging of the ear drum. In severe cases there is perforation of the eardrum, with mucopurulent discharge from the ear. In the past this often led to chronic suppurative otitis media, and even today, unless the condition is recognized and treated effectively, this may happen. Young children with otitis media seldom complain of earache, and as the signs of otitis are overshadowed by measles, the ears should be examined routinely.

(*b*) *Laryngitis.* Acute obstructive laryngitis (formerly called croup) may occasionally arise in the prodromal period, and is probably due to the direct action of the measles virus rather than to secondary infection. The intense inflammation and oedema of the larynx, vocal cords and epiglottis, tend to obstruct the airway. The clinical picture is striking with the onset of audible laryngeal stridor, and a hoarse squeaky cough and voice. In a more severe case, the child becomes restless and anxious, the respiratory movements are laboured with indrawing of the soft tissues of the root of the neck, lower intercostal and subcostal regions on inspiration. The appearance of cyanosis is the last and most dangerous sign. The lungs are usually clear on examination, and it is important not to confuse this condition with bronchitis or pneumonia.

(c) *Bronchitis.* In uncomplicated measles, there is a persistent cough, and occasional coarse rhonchi are heard in the lungs, but in established bronchitis, there is a rise in the respiratory rate, and widespread rhonchi and coarse crepitations are heard. Such a degree of involvement of the bronchi is an indication for antibiotic therapy.

(d) *Pneumonia.* The majority of cases are bronchopneumonic in type, and vary in severity from bronchiolitis, with a near normal chest X-ray, to cases having confluent areas of pneumonic consolidation. The condition arises at the height of the rash, presenting with an increase in cough, rapid distressed respiration and a tendency to cyanosis. The child is obviously ill, limp and prostrate. Widespread fine crepitations are heard over both lungs.

In a minority of cases, there is lobar pneumonia. This often appears later, as the rash is fading, with a recurrence of cough and fever, a rise in respiratory rate and, in older children, pleuritic pain. The usual clinical and radiological signs of lobar consolidations are found.

In both types of pneumonia, a wide range of microorganisms can be found in larnyngeal swabs or sputum, including *Strep. pneumoniae*, haemolytic streptococci, staphylococci and *Haemophilus influenzae.*

More than half the deaths in measles are due to pneumonia, and many of these are in children with pre-existing physical or mental defects, such as congenital heart disease or mongolism.

2 Central nervous system

(a) *Convulsions.* As with any acute febrile illness, convulsions may occur at the onset of the illness, especially in the 1–4 year age group.

(b) *Encephalitis.* This is an uncommon but important complication, which has an incidence of about one in 1000 cases.

Encephalitis occurs most commonly about 4–6 days after the appearance of the rash, usually at a time when the child is recovering normally. There is no association between the severity of the measles and the incidence of encephalitis. There is a return of fever with signs of meningeal irritation (headache, vomiting, neck and spinal rigidity). The child becomes drowsy, but this sometimes alternates with periods of noisy, unruly behaviour. In severe cases the drowsiness deepens to coma, and there may be convulsions and a variety of cranial nerve pareses. The coma may last from one or two days to several weeks. There may be an associated myelitis with spasticity of limbs, increased reflexes, extensor plantar responses, and retention of urine. Deep coma with dilated, sluggish pupils, is an ominous prognostic sign.

In most cases the CSF is abnormal, showing a lymphocytosis and raised protein but normal sugar levels. The EEG shows diffuse changes over the whole cortex.

There is a mortality of about 10 per cent and it is said that a considerable percentage of the survivors show some degree of mental or neurological impairment; however, in our experience the majority of the survivors, even where coma has lasted for a week or longer, appear to recover completely, as judged by clinical and EEG examination, and by the reports of parents and school teachers.

Minor indications of emotional instability, such as giggling or weeping, and residual spasticity may take several months to recover.

(c) *Subacute sclerosing panencephalitis* (*SSPE*). This is a rare form of encephalitis in children and adolescents, characterized by the insidious onset of mental deterioration and myoclonic fits, gradually progressing to generalized convulsions, coma and death. In recent years, it has been convincingly demonstrated that the disease is a late complication of measles, starting months or more usually several years after the attack of measles. The diagnosis is made by the typical picture and characteristic EEG changes, with a high measles antibody titre in the cerebrospinal fluid.

3   Miscellaneous

Rare complications include reactivation of primary tuberculosis, appendicitis and thrombocytopenic purpura.

Diagnosis

The combination of fever, catarrh, Koplik's spots and a rash, makes the diagnosis of measles a simple matter in most cases. A diagnosis in the prodromal stage is most often not made because of the failure to notice Koplik's spots. The rash may be confused with drug reactions, rubella, glandular fever, erythema multiforme, the rash of enterovirus infection, and even scarlet fever.

When laryngitis is an early feature, the possibility of laryngeal diphtheria or other causes of laryngeal obstruction should be considered.

There are no specific laboratory tests to establish the diagnosis; Turk cells are found in blood films, but these occur in other virus infections, especially rubella. Virological confirmation is possible in retrospect by the demonstration of rising antibody titres, but virus isolation in the acute stages of the illness is not generally available and remains a research procedure.

Prognosis

The mortality, which is very low, is almost entirely due to pneumonia or encephalitis. The former mortality of 80–100 deaths per year has fallen since the introduction of vaccination to 20–30 per year. A number of deaths are in children with severe physical or mental congenital defects.

Treatment

Cases of measles are nursed at home unless conditions are very poor or complications develop. The child usually refuses to eat in the acute stages, but adequate fluid intake is necessary. The patient's room should be warm and reasonably ventilated and visitors are kept to a minimum.

Prophylactic treatment with antibiotics should be reserved for 'poor risk' children.

Otitis media usually responds to penicillin or erythromycin treatment, and myringotomy is almost never necessary. In cases with perforation, the organism may be isolated from the discharge, and will give an accurate guide to further chemotherapy. It is important to follow up such cases until the ear drums and the hearing return to normal.

Acute obstructive laryngitis is best treated in hospital, the patient being nursed in an atmosphere of steam. Most cases will recover without surgical treatment, but deterioration, as shown by pallor, sweating, exhaustion, a PCO_2 level of 50 mm Hg or more, and above all cyanosis, necessitates tracheostomy.

Pneumonia complicating measles is associated with a variety of micro-organisms, but most cases respond to combined penicillin and streptomycin, or ampicillin. Severe cases, often staphylococcal, require the addition of cloxacillin. Cephaloridine is an effective alternative drug. Patients who are obviously limp and ill, or who show cyanosis, are nursed in an oxygen tent. A clear X-ray should be obtained before discharge.

The treatment of encephalitis is basically the medical and nursing care of an unconscious patient and includes:

1 Tube feeding to ensure an adequate caloric, protein and fluid intake.

2 Bladder catheterization to overcome retention of urine, and to measure the urinary output.

3 Regular checks of blood urea and electrolytes.

4 Frequent changes of position and intensive nursing care to prevent pressure sores.

5 Maintenance of a clear respiratory tract by nursing the patient in a prone or semi-prone position, by adequate physiotherapy to the chest, and by removal of all secretions by suction. Tracheostomy is occasionally necessary.

Corticosteroids have been recommended in encephalitis, and are said to promote rapid recovery. However, no satisfactory evidence exists to support this, and our personal experience of this form of treatment has been disappointing.

Prevention

During the febrile stage children are isolated as far as possible, although this does little to prevent infection in family contacts. Children return to school when they are clinically well, which usually entails at least a week of convalescence. Quarantine of school contacts is not necessary.

1 Passive immunization

Human normal immunoglobulin is an effective prophylactic but is in short supply. In general, its use is restricted to the protection of young children who are already ill at the time of exposure to measles and for the control of institutional outbreaks. Immunoglobulin is only effective when given during the first half of the incubation period. A dose of 500–750 mg will usually prevent an attack but the protection only lasts for 3–6 weeks.

2 Active immunization
Measles vaccination is now advocated on a community basis. A single dose of attenuated live-virus vaccine is advised for all children during the second year of life. The vaccine is stored in the freeze-dried state at domestic refrigerator temperature and is reconstituted with sterile water immediately before use and given by intramuscular injection. Most children have a short febrile reaction 7–10 days after the vaccination and about one third develop a rash, but these reactions are usually mild and acceptable. Rarely convulsions or very rarely encephalitis occur, but the incidence is much less than with natural measles. In children with (i) chronic heart or lung disease (ii) a history of convulsions or a family history of epilepsy and (iii) serious underdevelopment, it is desirable to modify a possible reaction to the vaccine by the simultaneous administration of human immunoglobulin with a specific measles antibody content.

Live measles vaccine is not given to children:
(i) Suffering from leukaemia, Hodgkin's disease or other lymphoma, or with impaired immunity mechanisms such as hypogammaglobulinaemia.
(ii) On treatment with corticosteroids, immunosuppressive drugs or X-ray therapy.
(iii) Suffering from any febrile illness, (other than a slight 'cold') untreated tuberculosis, or hypersensitivity to egg protein, polymyxin or neomycin.

The vaccine confers effective protection in about 90 per cent of children for at least 12 years, but the full duration of immunity is not yet known.

CHAPTER 10

Rubella

Rubella is a mild infectious disease, characterized by a discrete macular rash, and enlargement of the posterior cervical lymph glands. Rubella in a woman in early pregnancy causes damage to the fetus in a substantial percentage of cases and gives this otherwise trivial infection considerable importance.

Epidemiology

The causative virus may be isolated by tissue culture. The disease occurs throughout the world. There is increased prevalence in the spring and summer months. Cases occur sporadically with occasional localized epidemics. Every few years a more extensive epidemic spreads throughout several countries. It was after such an epidemic in 1940 that the occurrence of congenital defects in the babies of affected mothers was first noted.

Rubella is most frequently seen in school children and young adults. Recently it has been found that a considerable number of virologically proven cases gave no history of a rash. By adult life, 85 per cent of the population shows serological evidence of previous infection.

The disease spreads directly from case to case, by droplet infection. Infectivity lasts from about 5 days before to 5 days after the rash. Babies infected *in utero* can excrete the virus for months after birth and so cause further infections. Immunity is usually permanent, so that authentic second cases are rare.

Incubation period

Usually 17–18 days, but with limits of 14–21 days.

Clinical picture

Rubella is a mild illness. In young children the appearance of the rash may be the first sign of the disease. In older children and adults, there is usually a prodromal illness of about two days' duration or occasionally longer, with low-grade pyrexia, headache, general malaise, nasopharyngeal catarrh, sore throat and conjunctival irritation. Patients may notice tender swellings in the neck for several days before the appearance of the rash.

The rash, consisting of discrete macules, appears first on the face and neck, and spreads within 24 hours to the trunk and limbs. It fades after one or two days. The characteristic lymph gland enlargement particularly affects the posterior cervical groups which become palpable and tender, and persist for about a week. In some cases there is a generalized lymphadenopathy. In virologically proven cases, whoch have no rash, lymph gland enlargement is a more constant feature. Palpebral conjunctivitis is frequently found. The constitutional disturbance is usually slight and patients do not feel, or appear, particularly ill.

Complications
Serious complications of the clinical illness are almost unknown. A benign flitting polyarthritis may occur, and cases of post infectious encephalitis and thrombocytopenic purpura have occurred.

Rubella in a woman in the first four months of pregnancy may result in fetal damage. This complication is the single serious aspect of an otherwise innocuous disease. The fetal damage most commonly affects the eyes (cataract), the ears (perceptive deafness) and the heart (patent ductus arteriosus and septal defects). Occasionally the nervous system and the skeletal system are affected and hepatosplenomegaly and thrombocytopenic purpura may occur. Defects may be multiple and severe, and may result in abortion or stillbirth. More recently it has been found that the affected fetus may have persistent active infection for several months after birth, when the virus may be recovered from the urine or throat. Estimates of the incidence of fetal damage following maternal rubella vary, but average figures are shown in Table 3.

The greatest risk of fetal damage occurs before the mother knows she is pregnant. It may follow very mild and perhaps unrecognized attacks of rubella.

TABLE 3

Duration of pregnancy at time of infection	Percentage of cases suffering fetal damage ($\%$)
First 4 weeks	More than 50
4–8 weeks	About 25
8–12 weeks	About 10
12–16 weeks	About 5

Diagnosis
Rubella is most likely to be confused with mild attacks of glandular fever, measles, ECHO virus infection with a rash, and

drug sensitivity rashes. The white blood count shows a small percentage of Turk cells, and this may help to distinguish the condition from glandular fever. The virus can be isolated from the naso-pharynx by tissue culture. An accurate and rapid diagnosis is important in a pregnant woman and this is best achieved by demonstrating a rising antibody titre using the haemagglutination-inhibition technique. This may not be possible if the patient presents after the acute phase of the illness and in such cases, the demonstration of rubella-specific IgM (signifying recent infection) is a valuable test.

Fetal damage from rubella has to be distinguished from that due to congenital syphilis, toxoplasmosis, herpes simplex and cytomegalovirus infection.

Prognosis
There is virtually no mortality from rubella.

Treatment
There is no specific treatment, while symptomatic therapy only requires mild analgesics.

When a woman in the first four months of pregnancy develops an illness suggestive of rubella, the diagnosis should be confirmed serologically. If the diagnosis is confirmed, then therapeutic abortion will need to be considered, taking into account the duration of pregnancy at the time of infection, the social circumstances, and above all the attitude of the patient.

Prevention
No attempt need be made to isolate cases of rubella, particularly in school children, but pregnant women should avoid any exposure. There is no need to quarantine school contacts, and cases should return to school when the clinical symptoms have settled.

When a woman in early pregnancy is a close contact of rubella, serum is taken for antibody estimation. If the serum contains antibody (this will be true of 85 per cent of cases), the patient can be reassured that she will not contract the disease. In the 15 per cent of patients without antibody, it is important to watch for the development of clinical rubella and to confirm it virologically. Even in the absence of clinical illness, a further serum specimen should be examined in four weeks, to detect mild or subclinical infection. If rubella infection occurs even in subclinical form, therapeutic abortion would need consideration. There is no evidence that commercially available normal immunoglobulin affords any protection, even in large doses and is no longer recommended.

Active immunization

Rubella vaccination is recommended for all girls between their 11th and 14th birthdays. A previous history of rubella is not sufficiently reliable to justify withholding the vaccine. Two types of attenuated live-rubella vaccine are licensed for use in this country. 'Cendevax' (Cendehill strain) is the more attenuated and produces very few side-effects, but does not produce high antibody levels generally and in 5 per cent of patients produces none. The antibody levels produced may be boosted and prolonged by natural subclinical infection, but when this happens there may be a slight risk of fetal damage. 'Almevax' (RA 27 Popkin strain) is less attenuated and so produces higher and more prolonged antibody levels in virtually all cases, but at the cost of more frequent side-effects including sore throats, tender glands, rashes and joint pains.

A rational deployment of the two types of vaccine is to use Almevax in the routine childhood programme and to use Cendevax for the vaccination of selected groups of adult females. It is stored at 2–8°C (domestic refrigeration) and is used within an hour of reconstitution. Traces of vaccine virus are excreted in the nasopharynx of vaccinated persons, but controlled studies have failed to prove that infection is transmissible to susceptible contacts.

Vaccination is not offered routinely to women of childbearing age because of the possibility of damage to the fetus if pregnancy occurs within eight weeks. A woman who requests vaccination and is seronegative is vaccinated provided she agrees to avoid pregnancy for the following two months. A woman found to be seronegative in the antenatal period may be offered vaccination in the early post-partum period but it is not advisable to rely solely on the period of infertility which usually occurs then. The vaccine antibody response may be inhibited by blood transfusion at the time of delivery, but not by the earlier administration of anti-D immunoglobulin. In certain female groups such as school teachers, nursery staff, paediatric nurses,

C

obstetric unit and antenatal clinic staff, there may be special risks of contracting or disseminating rubella. Seronegative individuals in these groups should be vaccinated.

Rubella vaccination is contraindicated in the following circumstances:

1　Pregnancy.
2　Malignant conditions such as leukaemia or Hodgkin's disease.
3　Hypogammaglobulinaemia and other immunological deficiency states.
4　Corticosteroid or immunosuppressive drug treatment.
5　Vaccination is postponed if the patient is suffering from any febrile illness.

Cendevax is contraindicated in persons known to be hypersensitive to rabbit protein or neomycin. Almevax is contraindicated in neomycin or polymixin hypersensitivity. Because of the relatively early age at which vaccination is carried out, it will be several years before the true value of the vaccine in preventing fetal damage can be assessed. Two congenital rubella surveillance centres (a Southern Registry based on London and a Northern Registry based on Leeds) have been set up to evaluate progress.

CHAPTER 11

Mumps

Mumps is a generalized virus infection, causing localized inflamation of the salivary glands and occasionally complicated by orchitis, meningitis or pancreatitis.

Epidemiology

The causative virus may be readily isolated by tissue culture, and belongs to the paramyxovirus group. The source of infection is the saliva of a case, or an individual undergoing an inapparent infection. Transmission is by droplet infection, oral contact, or by articles recently contaminated by saliva. Infectivity lasts from a few days before the onset of salivary gland swelling, until the glands have completely regressed. Immunity is usually permanent, so that second attacks are rare. Mumps occurs throughout the world, and is endemic in Britain. Localized outbreaks appear from time to time, particularly in residential institutions. The disease principally affects school children and young adults. There is a slight increase of incidence in the spring.

Incubation period
This is usually 17–19 days, with limits of 12–28 days.

Clinical picture
Mumps may present with generalized features, such as headache, vomiting, sore throat and pyrexia, lasting for one or two days before signs of salivary gland involvement appear. However, in many cases salivary gland inflammation is the first sign of the illness. The parotid glands are most commonly involved and parotitis is usually heralded by discomfort and tenderness at the angle of the jaw, aggravated by chewing. Occasionally there is redness at the opening of the parotid duct in the mouth. The parotitis may be unilateral, but is more often bilateral, and usually one gland is affected after the other at an interval of 1–5 days. In a minority of cases the submandibular glands are involved, occasionally alone, but usually along with the parotids. Each gland is enlarged for several days before it gradually subsides, so that the whole illness may last from one to two weeks. The glands are tender, but not often painful and the overlying skin is not reddened. When several glands are involved the flow of saliva is reduced, and the mouth becomes dry. The temperature is raised at the onset, and there are often exacerbations of fever as other glands enlarge. The pyrexia settles, often abruptly, as the glands regress.

Occasionally the disease presents only as a benign viral meningitis; more rarely, only as an architis or pancreatitis, without salivary gland involvement. In a minority of cases, mumps remains clinically inapparent and this is of considerable importance in the spread of the disease.

Complications

1 Genito-urinary tract

Orchitis is the most common complication and occurs in about 20 per cent of post-pubertal males. It is usually unilateral and often appears as the other signs of illness are settling. There is an abrupt return of fever and malaise, with the rapid development of a red painful swelling of the testis, which lasts for several days before gradually subsiding. In severe cases, gradual atrophy of the affected testis may occur in the ensuing months. In severe bilateral orchitis, such atrophy may lead to sterility, but this is very rare. When orchitis is the only feature of mumps, it must be distinguished from bacterial orchitis secondary to a urinary tract infection, and from acute torsion of the testis.

In the female, oophoritis occurs much less frequently and is usually mild. Rare complications include prostatitis in the male and mastitis in the female.

2 Central nervous system

Neurological complications may occur at any time in the illness and are more common in older children and adults.

(a) Clinically inapparent meningeal involvement in mumps is very common as can be shown by CSF examination in uncomplicated cases.

Clinical meningitis is common and presents with fever, headache and vomiting with neck and spinal rigidity. This is a benign condition but is often miscalled 'mumps encephalitis' wrongly suggesting a more serious condition. The CSF shows a considerably raised lymphocyte count of 200 to 2000 cells and a moderately raised protein. Mumps virus can be isolated from the CSF in most cases. This may be the only manifestation of mumps infection and virological surveys have shown it to be the second most common cause of viral meningitis, after entero-viral infections.

(b) Encephalitis, with or without meningitis does occur after mumps, but it is a very rare and serious condition, occasionally fatal. This presents with disturbed behaviour, altered levels of consciousness or coma and sometimes spastic weakness. It is similar to the other forms of encephalitis, such as occurs after measles.

(c) Involvement of the nerves of the inner ear is rare, but may result in permanent deafness, partial or complete in one or both ears.

(d) Other rare neurological manifestations include myelitis and polyneuritis, sometimes called 'paralytic mumps'.

3 Pancreas

Acute pancreatitis is an uncommon complication presenting with fever, vomiting, upper abdominal pain and tenderness. Unlike other forms of pancreatitis, a raised serum amylase has little diagnostic value, as this is raised in uncomplicated parotitis. A raised serum lipase level would be better confirmatory evidence, but this test is not generally available. Mumps pancreatitis is usually benign and settles in a few days and there is no conclusive evidence that diabetes follows this condition.

Diagnosis

In a typical case, the diagnosis is simple, but atypical and mild cases are common and may cause difficulty. In parotitis, the angle of the jaw is obscured and difficult to define, whereas in lymph gland or other swellings of the neck, the angle is clearly palpable.

Mumps parotitis must be distinguished from other causes of parotid swelling all of which are rare in children:

1 Acute suppurative parotitis—this is most common in the elderly debilitated patient. In the early stages, there is redness of the skin over the swelling (which is absent in mumps) and later, abscess formation is common.

2 Salivary duct calculi—the swelling is intermittent and unilateral.

3 Sarcoidosis—the parotitis is bilateral and subacute, and there is often evidence of uveal tract involvement.

4 Parotid tumours.

5 Sjörgren's syndrome—subacute parotitis in association with rheumatoid arthritis.

In difficult cases, the diagnosis may be confirmed by the isolation of mumps virus from the saliva or urine, and by the demonstration of a rise in serum antibody. Two antibodies are formed in the serum, the S-type (Soluble) which appears and disappears quickly and the V-type (Virus) which appears more slowly and persists for long periods.

Prognosis
Apart from a very rare death from encephalomyelitis, there is no
mortality from mumps. Permanent sterility or deafness are very
rare sequelae.

Treatment
This is symptomatic, and consists of mild analgesics, mouth
washes and the provision of a fluid or easily-chewed diet. Cases
remain at home while symptoms last. Bed rest is unnecessary in
children and females, but is advisable in males until the
temperature settles. A short course of corticosteroids may
reduce the period of pain and swelling in orchitis, but there is
no evidence that steroids prevent the late atrophy of the testis.

Prevention
Isolation of cases does little to prevent the spread of the disease
in the community, and quarantine of contacts is not necessary.
Normal human immunoglobulin does not usually confer passive
immunity against mumps. It is possible to prepare an effective
hyperimmune gammaglobulin, but as there is little or no
practical application for this, it has never been made generally
available. An effective vaccination using a live-attenuated vaccine is advocated in the United States and the Soviet Union
but a survey of the complications of mumps in Britain con-
cluded that routine vaccination would not be justified.

CHAPTER 12

Viral Hepatitis

Viral hepatitis is a common infectious disease, characterized by
diffuse inflammatory changes in the liver. The clinical illness
presents as a febrile systemic upset with gastrointestinal symptoms followed in many cases by jaundice.
   Viral hepatitis generally occurs in two distinct types differing
in mode of transmission, incubation period, clinical severity,

mortality and serological findings. The more common type is hepatitis A or infective hepatitis (sometimes called epidemic hepatitis or short-incubation hepatitis). The less common but more severe type is hepatitis B or serum hepatitis (sometimes called long-incubation hepatitis).

Hepatitis may occur in the course of glandular fever, cytomegalovirus infections and, very rarely, in a wide variety of other virus diseases, e.g. herpes simplex, entero and adenovirus infections. Yellow fever is a severe type of viral hepatitis occurring in the tropics and caused by an arbovirus.

Only hepatitis A and B will be dealt with in this chapter.

In recent years, there have been a number of cases of hepatitis (including post-transfusion hepatitis) not related to hepatitis A or B virus, cytomegalovirus or Epstein–Barr virus infection and it is likely that such cases are due to other as yet unidentified viruses. These are referred to as nonA nonB hepatitis.

Epidemiology

Hepatitis A

Hepatitis A virus (HAV) has now been positively identified. It is a small virus, 25–28 mm in diameter and can be demonstrated by immune electronmicroscopy in the faeces of patients with hepatitis A; similar virus particles have been seen in the tissues of animals experimentally infected with this virus. Antibodies to this virus can also be demonstrated in the serum of patients recovering from hepatitis A. These tests are not yet available outside research laboratories and much of the information so far available about the spread of infection, period of infectivity, carrier state and immunity has been obtained from the study of the natural disease and from experimental infection in human volunteers.

The natural disease appears only in human hosts but chimpanzees and marmosets can be infected with hepatitis A virus experimentally. Transmission generally takes place by contact with infected faeces, either through direct person to person contact or through contaminated water, or food giving rise to explosive outbreaks. Infectivity precedes the first symptoms by several days and is generally considered to persist for a week or so after the appearance of jaundice. Anicteric and subclinical cases are quite common and are an important factor in the spread of the disease.

The disease is endemic in Britain. Explosive local epidemics, probably foodborne, have occurred particularly in institutions such as boarding schools and army camps. During the Second World War, infective hepatitis was the main medical problem in the British Army in the Middle East. There is a seasonal increase of the disease in the autumn and winter. Cases mostly occur among school children and young adults. Travellers to highly endemic areas in North Africa, the Middle East and the Indian subcontinent are at greater risk if they bypass the ordinary tourist routes. Lasting immunity seems to follow an attack.

Hepatitis B

In hepatitis B virus (HBV) infection, three distinct morphological forms can be demonstrated in the serum by electronmicroscopy: a small spherical particle 20 mm in diameter, a tubular form of the same diameter and a larger spherical particle of 42 mm in diameter. The latter is named the Dane particle which is the causal virus itself, possessing a surface coat and an inner core. The smaller particles probably represent the broken-down surface coating of the larger Dane particle and their detection by haemagglutination or radioimmunoassay is an important step in the diagnosis of hepatitis B or the carrier state. This hepatitis B surface antigen (HB_sAg) was formerly called Australia Antigen or hepatitis associated antigen (HAA). Antibodies develop later in the infection to both surface (HB_sAB) and core antigen (HB_cAB) and whereas HB_sAB antibody usually disappears within months, core antibody lasts much longer and may provide a marker of past infection. It is now possible to subtype the surface antigen of which two forms exist, namely ad and ay; although their relationship to virulence remains uncertain, subtyping may be useful epidemiologically.

A third antigen distinct from both surface and core antigen has been found recently in some HB_sAg positive sera. Evidence suggests that this antigen, designated 'e' may be a marker for higher infectivity and its persistence may indicate the possible development of chronic liver disease.

The main route of transmission is parenteral through transfusion of infected blood or blood products: the use of contaminated syringes and needles, dental or medical instruments or other parenteral means, such as tattooing, acupuncture, ear-piercing or even sharing a razor. The use of disposable syringes and needles has greatly reduced transmission by contaminated syringes except in drug addicts where infection is increasingly common. The amount of blood necessary to transmit infection is very small but not all people receiving infected blood develop jaundice and anicteric hepatitis is probably common. Other body fluids such as saliva and semen may contain the infective agent leading to transmission by oral or sexual routes; male homosexuals appear to be particularly at risk. It has been estimated that approximately one per cent of the population of this country are asymptomatic carriers of hepatitis B virus. In some tropical countries the carriage rate may be very high and transmission through insect bites has been postulated. The disease is generally sporadic, occurring mainly in urban adults and older teenagers, although it may be widespread among mentally subnormal children in certain institutions. In the past, there have been a number of severe outbreaks in renal dialysis units but the adoption of strict precautionary measures has led to a drastic reduction in such cases. There is no demonstrable cross-immunity between hepatitis A and B and this is reflected in the ability of normal human immunoglobulin to prevent hepatitis A but not hepatitis B.

HB_sAg generally disappears from the blood within a month of the onset of the disease but occasionally persists for much longer periods and such patients may go on to develop chronic liver disease. Patients with chronic renal failure. Down's syndrome and those receiving immunosuppressive treatment frequently carry HB_sAg for long periods.

Pathology

This is identical in both types and is well recognized from liver biopsy. There is a centrilobular cell necrosis and a mononuclear cell infiltration of the whole organ. The basic structural framework of the liver is preserved so that cellular replacement and complete recovery takes place. Rarely in severe cases, there is a massive hepatocellular necrosis, with disruption of the hepatic architecture leading to post-necrotic scarring in the survivors.

C*

Incubation period

In hepatitis A this is on average 28 days with limits of 2–6 weeks.

In hepatitis B this is on average 100 days with limits of 6 weeks to 6 months.

Clinical picture

In hepatitis A the onset is usually abrupt with fever, aching limbs, upper abdominal discomfort, anorexia, nausea and vomiting. Smoking becomes distasteful. Severe abdominal pain is not a feature of hepatitis, although mild pain may be present. The fever settles in a few days, while digestive symptoms and lassitude persist. After a varying period of 3–6 days or occasionally longer, the urine becomes dark, the faeces pale and clinical jaundice appears. The jaundice lasts for about a week in an average case, although it may range from only a few days in mild cases to several weeks in severe cases. With the appearance of the jaundice, the symptoms usually abate and the appetite begins to return. Pruritis is troublesome in a few cases. The disease tends to be milder in children and more severe in adults, particularly middle-aged or pregnant women.

In hepatitis B, the onset is usually insidious with anorexia, vague upper abdominal discomfort and nausea progressing gradually to jaundice. Fever may be absent or mild. Transient arthralgia or even frank arthritis and an urticarial rash may develop but otherwise the clinical picture is broadly similar with hepatitis A.

The usual clinical findings are jaundice, a slow pulse and a smoothly enlarged liver which may be a little tender. Occasionally the spleen is palpably enlarged.

Complications

1   Relapsing hepatitis

In about 10 per cent of cases, there is a relapse of the disease, either during the icteric period or shortly afterwards. Occasionally the relapse is more severe and protracted than the original illness.

2   Cholestatic hepatitis

In some cases, the level of bilirubin rises and pruritis develops, after the other liver function tests have returned to normal levels. This state persists for weeks or even months, and is due to intrahepatic cholestasis which will eventually clear spontaneously. When the patient is seen for the first time at this stage, the condition may be extremely difficult to differentiate from other causes of obstructive jaundice—either intrahepatic or extrahepatic.

3   Post-hepatitis syndrome

When the jaundice has faded, the patient soon returns to normal health, but in a minority of cases, upper abdominal discomfort, dyspepsia and lassitude may recur from time to time for a period of weeks or months, particularly after severe physical exertion. This is not associated with organic liver disease and liver function tests as well as liver biopsy will show no abnormality.

4   Fulminant hepatitis

A rare but very serious complication is massive hepatic necrosis. This presents as drowsiness and mental confusion, progressing to coma, after jaundice has been present for several days. In addition to the usual evidence of a severe hepatitis, there is aminoaciduria and a falling blood urea level. When coma is established, the outcome is usually fatal.

5   Chronic hepatatitis

This is defined as continuing hepatitis of at least six months' duration as demonstrated by liver function tests and liver biopsy.

Two varieties can be recognized: chronic persistent hepatitis and chronic active hepatitis (also known as chronic aggressive hepatitis).

(i)   Chronic persistent hepatatis is characterized by modestly raised serum aminotransferase, slight bilirubinaemia, continuing fatigue and discomfort over the liver. Liver biopsy shows inflammation confined to the portal zones with little hepatocellular necrosis. It may follow a typical attack of acute viral hepatitis of either type but may also be due to drugs, alcoholic excess or chronic inflammatory bowel disease. It has a good prognosis and settles without treatment.

(ii)   In chronic active hepatitis, the clinical and biochemical abnormalities are more pronounced and histologically inflammation extends beyond the portal zone into the hepatic parenchyma. Some of the cases undoubtedly follow hepatitis B but follow up studies of hepatitis A outbreaks have shown little evidence of the later development of chronic active hepatitis. Other causes include drugs, autoimmune hepatitis and Wilson's disease. There is progressive hepatocellular dysfunction leading ultimately to hepatic failure. Although corticosteroids appear to be beneficial in autoimmune chronic hepatitis, their value in HB$_s$Ag associated cases remains doubtful.

6 Neonatal hepatitis
Hepatitis B virus is one of the causes of neonatal hepatitis and evidence suggests that a newborn baby is more liable to develop this if the mother develops acute hepatitis B during pregnancy than if she is an asymptomatic carrier.

Diagnosis
In the pre-icteric period, hepatitis may be confused with many general infections, or even with acute surgical conditions of the abdomen. Non-icteric cases are usually diagnosed as the result of the occurrence of jaundice in a contact.

Jaundiced cases have to be distinguished from the many other causes of jaundice, such as:

1 Infective conditions. (a) Causing hepatitis, such as glandular fever and leptospirosis, (b) causing haemolysis and jaundice, such as Gram-negative septicaemias.

2 Drug-induced jaundice, which can be produced in two main ways.

(a) A drug-sensitivity reaction producing an intrahepatic cholestatic jaundice may follow the use of chlorpromazine, PAS, sulphonamides or erythromycin estofolate. Apart from the jaundice, there may be fever, lymphadenopathy and eosinophilia. Certain androgens and some birth control pills may also produce cholestatic jaundice. The jaundice is of the obstructive type and the liver is often enlarged. The jaundice is usually reversible when the drug is withdrawn, and corticosteroids have little effect.

(b) Less commonly by direct liver cell damage, with such drugs as pyrazinamide, halothane, paracetamol, isoniazid, rifampicin, monoamine-oxidase inhibitors and certain organic poisons. These produce a hepatitis very similar clinically and biochemically to viral hepatitis. Alcohol can produce both hepatocellular as well as cholestatic jaundice.

3 Obstructive jaundice due to gall-bladder disease or neoplasm. In jaundice due to gall-stone obstruction, severe pain may be a diagnostic feature. Differentiation is more difficult when cholecystitis or cholangitis is present.

Laboratory tests

Urine tests and liver function tests may help to distinguish the obstructive from the toxic or infective type of jaundice.

In hepatitis, urobilinogen appears in excess in the urine before the appearance of jaundice (Ehrlichs aldehyde test). When jaundice appears, urobilinogen disappears, but bilirubin appears in the urine (Fouchers test or Ictotest Tablet test). In obstructive jaundice, bilirubin appears in the urine from the onset.

Apart from the level of bilirubin, the two most valuable liver function tests are:

1 *Serum aminotransferases*—particularly serum alanine aminotransferase or SALT (formerly called serum glutamic pyruvic transaminase or SGPT). This enzyme is released into the blood in excess when liver cell necrosis is taking place. The normal level is below 50 units. In viral hepatitis, the level rises, even before jaundice is present, to several hundred units. In the first week of jaundice, the level rises to about 500–1500 units; in the second week, drops to about 200–300 units, and in the following week or two returns to normal. In obstructive jaundice, the SALT is barely raised at the onset, but rises slowly to about 200 units over a period of several weeks.

2 *Serum alkaline phosphatase.* The enzyme is formed in the bones and liver and is removed from the blood by the liver and excreted in the bile. The normal level is below 15 King–Armstrong units. In viral hepatitis, the level rises slightly but is not usually above 35 units. In obstructive jaundice, the level is often higher at 40–80 units.

Flocculation tests (thymol turbidity, colloidal gold, etc.). These tests reflect minor changes in the globulin pattern. In viral hepatitis, they often become strongly positive and may remain so for several weeks, even after the jaundice has settled. In obstructive jaundice, the tests seldom become positive. These tests are significantly less sensitive than the enzyme tests and are no longer used routinely in many hospitals.

The liver function tests will be most helpful in distinguishing the types of jaundice in the first two or three weeks of illness, but after four or five weeks the results may become equivocal. The most consistent change is the high aminotransferase level (SALT) in the early stages of viral hepatitis.

In viral hepatitis, the differential white cell count shows a leucopenia with a relative lymphocytosis.

Cholecystography or intravenous cholangiography is seldom successful in the presence of jaundice, but a plain X-ray of the abdomen is useful, as gall stones may be seen.

When jaundice persists and the clinical picture and liver function tests suggest obstructive jaundice, radioactive liver scan, ultrasonography and needle biopsy are useful procedures but laparotomy is often necessary to reach a diagnosis.

Prognosis
Hepatitis A is normally benign and complete recovery takes place. The mortality is about 0·1 per cent of jaundiced cases and death is usually due to massive hepatic necrosis with coma, most commonly occurring in middle-aged women. In hepatitis B the mortality is always higher and hospital epidemics have occurred in recent years with an exceptional mortality of 20 per cent or higher. Hepatitis results in 200–300 deaths annually.

Treatment
In the uncomplicated case, a period of rest is usual until the symptoms and jaundice have settled, and the urine is free of bile, although strict bed rest is not necessary. Routine serum bilirubin and aminotransferase estimations can be a useful guide to progress. Food intake will be dictated by the patient's appetite, and particular foods, such as fat or eggs, are not prohibited. The diet should contain as high a calorie content as the patient will tolerate. Convalescence should not be hurried, and alcohol and severe exercise should be avoided for several months after hepatitis.

In cases of massive liver necrosis with coma, the conventional medical treatment is protein-free high carbohydrate intravenous feeding with oral neomycin to sterilize the gut, but this does not appear to influence the fatal course of the disease and corticosteroid treatment is similarly of little value. Recovery in occasional patients in the younger age groups has been reported following the use of charcoal haemoperfusion or haemodialysis using polyacrylonitrile membrane and a great deal of active research continues in this field.

Jaundice due to intrahepatic cholestasis may persist for many weeks or months after other evidence of active infection has settled, and corticosteroids may cause satisfactory clearing, thereby avoiding the prospect of liver biopsy or laparotomy.

Prevention

Hepatitis A

At present, isolation of cases in hospital or at home does little to prevent the spread of this disease. School contacts are not normally quarantined, but mild unexplained malaise among contacts should lead to exclusion from school. In a school or institutional outbreak, individual or paper towels should be used. Normal human immunoglobulin is of proved value in preventing the disease in contacts, and is advocated in special circumstances such as outbreaks in institutions. It is given by intramuscular injection in a dose of 250 mg for young children and 500 mg for those over 10 years and is effective when given in the two weeks after exposure. Travellers can also be protected for up to 6 months, by a dose of 750 mg.

Hepatitis B

Preventive measures are concerned with the safer selection and handling of blood in medical technology and include:

1 Blood donors are not accepted with a history of jaundice or hepatitis in the previous 12 months, or if they have been in house contact with hepatitis or received a transfusion of blood or blood products in the previous six months. Donors are now routinely screened for HB_sAg and excluded if positive. Those with negative HB_sAg but positive surface antibody are accepted for production of specific anti-hepatitis B immunoglobulin.

2 The preparation of blood products from 'small pools' of blood.

3 The use of individually sterilized or disposable syringes and needles for all injections, including mass immunization campaigns and dentistry. Registered drug addicts should be instructed in the proper care of syringes.

4 Precautions in laboratories are necessary, including the use of automatic 'no-touch' equipment, screw-top containers, protective clothing and disposable equipment.

5 Special precautions are necessary in renal dialysis units, including the screening of patients and staff for hepatitis B antigen, the use of protective gloves and clothing, disposable elements in kidney machines and the avoidance of blood for priming machines or transfusion whenever possible.

6 Contaminated articles should be heat sterilized or incine-

rated. Liquid disinfectants are unreliable, although hypochlorite and glutaraldehyde solutions are the most useful.

7   A limited amount of specific anti-hepatitis B immunoglobulin is available for the protection of hospital staff. It is used in the case of accidental inoculation of infected blood but the value is not yet known.

CHAPTER 13

Viral Infections of the Nervous System

Infection of the nervous system may be caused by a wide variety of microorganisms, including protozoa (malaria and toxoplasmosis), fungae (torulosis), spirochaetes (syphilis and leptospirosis), and various bacteria and viruses. This chapter deals with known or presumed viral infections, as summarized in Table 4.

1   Viral meningitis

This is a benign self-limiting disease which may be caused by a variety of viruses. Coxsackie and ECHO viruses are responsible for localized epidemics in the summer months, and mumps virus causes many sporadic cases. Children, particularly boys, and young adults are mainly affected. The onset is sudden with fever, headache, vomiting and signs of neck and spinal rigidity. The cerebrospinal fluid is abnormal, with a raised protein (0·5–1 g/litre), a raised white cell count, mostly lymphocytes (50–500 cells/mm^3) and a normal sugar. The isolation of virus from the CSF is unusual except in mumps infection, but is diagnostic; otherwise the aetiology may be confirmed by rising antibody titres in paired sera and by the isolation of the virus from the throat or faeces. Cases recover completely with symptomatic treatment and there is no mortality.

A clinically similar illness occurs in leptospirosis (canicola fever).

TABLE 4

Organism	Disease	Comments
Arbovirus Eastern & Western Equine Venezuelan Japanese B Murray Valley St Louis Russian Spring—Summer	Epidemic encephalitis in foreign countries	Transmitted from host animal to man, by mosquitoes, mites, etc.
Louping Ill	Encephalitis (rare)	An infection of sheep in Scotland and Northern England.
Enterovirus Poliomyelitis (1, 2 & 3)	Poliomyelitis	Viral meningitis common. Occasional encephalitis
Coxsackie (A & B) ECHO	Epidemic viral meningitis	Paralytic disease very rare.
Herpesvirus Herpesvirus hominis	Encephalitis	Occasional viral meningitis.
Varicella-zoster (V.Z.)	Post-infectious meningo-encephalo- myelitis (uncommon)	
Herpesvirus simiae	Fatal encephalitis	Transmitted by monkey bite.
Cytomegalovirus	Neurological dis- ease in infancy	Occasional polyneuritis.
Paramyxovirus Mumps	Viral meningitis	Occasional encephalo- myelitis.
Measles	Post-infectious meningo-encephalo- myelitis (uncommon)	
Other viruses Rabies	Fatal encephalitis	Transmitted by animal bites.
Lymphocytic chlorio- meningitis	Viral meningitis (rare)	

2 Viral encephalitis

The following types of encephalitis occur:
(a) Epidemic encephalitis (arbovirus).
(b) Sporadic encephalitis (presumed viral).
(c) Post-infectious meningo-encephalomyelitis.
(d) Epidemic myalgic encephalitis.
(e) Subacute sclerosing panencephalitis (SSPE).
(f) Epidemic encephalitis lethargica.

Epidemic encephalitis (arbovirus). Outbreaks of encephalitis due to a variety of arboviruses occur in many parts of the world, particularly Japan, Russia, South America, Australia and the USA. The mortality of most types is 10–20 per cent and neurological or psychological sequelae occur in some survivors. The only type which occurs in Britain is 'Louping Ill' which is largely confined to sheep-rearing areas, such as the Scottish borders; this disease is common among sheep and is occasionally conveyed to shepherds by the sheep tick. It has also occurred in abattoir and laboratory workers.

Sporadic encephalitis. Approximately half the reported cases of encephalitis are of a sporadic nature. Herpes simplex virus is responsible for a proportion of these cases and enteroviruses account for a few, but in the majority of cases no aetiological agent can be identified. The actual proportion of herpetic cases is not known, as brain biopsy may be necessary to establish this diagnosis. The mortality of this type varies from 20 to 60 per cent in different series. Treatment is unsatisfactory and is largely the support of vital functions and the use of dexamethasone to reduce intracerebral pressure. It is accepted that the older antiviral drugs (idoxuridine and cytosine arabinoside) are without value. The newer antiviral drug adenine arabinoside is now being advocated but as yet there is no convincing evidence of its effectiveness.

Post-infectious meningo-encephalomyelitis. This is an uncommon complication of certain virus infections such as measles, chickenpox and mumps, and a rare complication of influenza, rubella and vaccinia. The illness usually occurs about 10 days after the onset of the viral infection, but virus has never been recovered from the brain except rarely in measles encephalitis. A similar illness occurred after the use of nerve tissue-containing rabies vaccine. Treatment is supportive and there is little evidence that corticosteroids are of value. The mortality varies with the original virus infection, being about 50 per cent in vaccinia; 10 per cent following measles and less in the other diseases. There are occasionally serious sequelae in survivors.

Epidemic myalgic encephalomyelitis. This condition has been described in a number of postwar epidemics mainly affecting hospital nursing staff in Britain and elsewhere. The onset is insidious with depression, difficulty in concentration, parasthesiae, irregular sensory changes and occasional spastic weakness in the limbs. Myalgic pain is common in the trunk and limb muscles. The CSF is normal, and no virus has been isolated from cases. There is no mortality, but fatigue and emotional lability persist in some cases for many months.

Subacute sclerosing panencephalitis (SSPE). This is a rare subacute type of encephalitis occurring months or more usually several years after an attack of measles. There is slowly progressive mental and neurological deterioration leading to a fatal outcome. A high level of measles antibody is found in the CSF and measles virus has been found in the brain.

Epidemic encephalitis lethargica. A world-wide epidemic of severe encephalitis affected Britain in the years 1918–26. The mortality rate was about 50 per cent and many of the survivors developed progressive psychotic states and Parkinsonism. No virological studies were possible at the time, and there is no convincing evidence that the disease still occurs.

Clinical features

The onset of encephalitis is usually acute with fever, headache, vomiting, irritability and photophobia. There may be fluctuation in the level of consciousness and changes in the personality with confused and abnormal behaviour. As the illness develops, the patient usually becomes progressively more drowsy and disturbed and eventually comatose. Involuntary movements, twitching or frank convulsions are common. In post-infectious encephalitis, evidence of myelitis is frequently present with spasticity of the legs and retention of urine. In herpes simplex cases focal signs such as hemiplegia or aphasia are common, but are unusual in other types.

The CSF usually shows a raised protein and lymphocyte count. The electroencephalogram usually shows a diffuse slow-wave pattern without any focal features, although the latter are common in herpes simplex cases.

Differential diagnosis

The following important conditions, most of which require urgent treatment, must be distinguished from viral meningitis and encephalitis.

(a) Tuberculous meningitis. The clinical picture may not be dissimilar and it is vitally important to exclude tuberculous meningitis first. A truly equivocal case should receive anti-tuberculous treatment.

(b) Partially-treated acute bacterial meningitis.

(c) Neurological involvement in syphilis, toxoplasmosis and malaria.

(d) Cerebrovascular disease, including subdural haematoma and subarachnoid haemorrhage.

(e) Space-occupying lesions, including abscess, aneurysm and tumour.

(f) Drug overdose and chemical poisoning (including lead).

A number of microbiological and biochemical tests on the blood and CSF may be necessary to establish the diagnosis and in difficult cases special investigations may be necessary, including electroencephalography (EEG), radioactive scanning of the brain, computer-assisted tomography, cerebral angiography and brain biopsy.

3 Acute infective polyneuritis (Guillain–Barré syndrome)

This is a rare sporadic disease of adults and older children, long suspected of being of viral origin. In some cases, cytomegalovirus has been isolated from the urine or throat, with a high or rising antibody titre in the blood. Polyneuritis is a rare complication of glandular fever and may also occur in other Epstein–Barr viral infections without a glandular fever-like illness. Influenca vaccines have been incriminated in the United States.

There is often a preceding upper respiratory infection and sore throat, followed in about a week by the onset of symmetrical flaccid paralysis of the limbs and trunk, and symmetrical sensory loss in the distal parts of the limbs. This paralysis may extend to involve the muscles of respiration in severe cases. In addition there may be facial paralysis and bulbar involvement with difficulty in swallowing and coughing. The disease must be distinguished from poliomyelitis and diphtheritic polyneuritis. The CSF shows the striking abnormality of a greatly raised protein, often more than 3 g/litre, without any rise in the white cell count.

The paralysis recovers completely, although severe cases may require up to two years. Physiotherapy is necessary to prevent deformity. Corticosteroids have been strongly recommended in the past, but are now considered to be of very doubtful value. Respiratory failure requires tracheotomy and assisted ventilation in a specialized artificial respiration unit.

4   Reye's syndrome

An encephalopathic illness in which a previously healthy child develops convulsions and fever and quickly lapses into status epilepticus. The liver enlarges rapidly and there may be evidence of hepatic failure. The condition is frequently fatal. The CSF remains normal throughout except for a low sugar. Though frequently confused with encephalitis, autopsy shows only a swollen brain with no histological evidence of encephalitis. The liver shows fatty degeneration. The cause remains unknown but an association with various virus infections has been noted. Present evidence suggests that the disease although uncommon may occur more frequently than previously supposed.

CHAPTER 14

Rabies

This is a viral zoonosis, transmitted to man by the bite of an infected animal.

Epidemiology

Rabies virus belongs to the rhabdovirus group. The disease occurs in every continent except Australia. In Europe rabies has moved slowly from Poland into Germany and France over the last 30 years. The red fox is the main vector in Europe, but other mammals may carry and transmit the disease. In Asia dogs and wolves are the main vectors and in South America it is the vampire bat. The dog and to a lesser extent the cat are usually the final links in the chain of infection leading to the human case. Animals are normally only infectious for a period of about two weeks as they become ill and die with rabies: the main exception is the vampire bat which is a healthy carrier. In animals, rabies occurs in two main forms (a) 'furious' rabies (dogs, cats) the animal becomes excited and aggressive, runs away out of control and bites anything in its path (b) 'dumb' rabies (foxes) the animal becomes lethargic and tame, and may approach humans, often appearing frightened, cringing and partially paralysed.

Human disease almost invariably results from an animal bite or scratch; case-to-case spread in humans is almost unknown.

Britain has been free of rabies for several decades, although a number of animals in quarantine kennels develop the disease. Human rabies occurs in Britain as an imported infection from time to time, but is not capable of further spread.

Incubation period
This is usually 2–8 weeks, but with limits of 10 days to 2 years. Incubation tends to be short in children and in bites on the head and neck.

Clinical picture
The first symptom is often discomfort and parasthesiae at the site of the bite. This is followed by fever, headache, malaise and an anxious personality change. Painful contraction of smooth muscle in the pharynx may lead to fear of swallowing and excessive salivation. A similar mechanism may lead to painful and difficult micturition. As the disease progresses there is increasing personality change with periods of excitability, fear and anxiety. Terminal flaccid paralysis is common.

Diagnosis
The disease must be distinguished from encephalitis, tetanus and poliomyelitis. The diagnosis may be confirmed post mortem by the:
(i)   demonstration of antigen in brain tissue by immunofluorescence,
(ii) microscopic demonstration of Negri bodies in the brain,
(iii) isolation of rabies virus by mouse inoculation.

Prognosis

Rabies is always fatal. There have been isolated reports of recovery but in each case the disease may have been modified by previous vaccination.

Treatment

This is symptomatic to relieve pain and anxiety and to attempt the support of vital functions. Although the risk to attendant staff is very slight, it is recommended that the patient should be strictly isolated and that staff wear goggles, masks and gloves in addition to being vaccinated.

Prevention

Vaccination

Human diploid cell vaccine (Merieux vaccine) is a killed virus preparation and is now the only vaccine in use. It is more potent and safer than the older duck embryo and Semple's rabbit brain vaccines which are no longer used.

(i) *Pre-exposure vaccination*—the course is 1 ml intramuscularly, repeated in 1 month and boosted in 1 year with repeat boost doses at 2- to 3-year intervals. Reactions are rare and mild and there are no contra-indications.

(ii) *Post-exposure management*—when a person is bitten by an animal in a known rabies area, if possible the biting animal is secured and kept for 10 days. In most cases an infected animal will develop rabies within this period and post-mortem will confirm the diagnosis. If the animal remains well after 10–14 days it is highly unlikely but not impossible that it has rabies.

Because of the long incubation period, it is normally possible to vaccinate a bitten patient and so prevent the disease developing. The vaccine is given at days 1, 3, 7, 14, 30 and 90 and if possible serum antibodies are estimated at day 30. If the bite is large, particularly in the head or neck region or more important, if the animal is proved to be rabid, hyperimmune antirabies immunoglobulin (Hyper-rab) is given in addition in a dose of 20 units/kg body weight. Most of the dose is given intramuscularly but about a third is infiltrated into the wound.

Further public health preventive measures are summarized as follows:

1　To prevent rabid animals from entering Britain
(a)　propaganda and legal penalties to prevent smuggling of animals,
(b)　quarantine of all legally-imported animals for one year,
(c)　facilities to confirm the diagnosis of suspected animal rabies are available in the Veterinary Pathology Laboratory, Weybridge, Surrey.
2　To prepare for animal rabies entering Britain
(a)　contingency plans to deal with an outbreak, involving police, vets and environmental staff,
(b)　vaccination of all categories of staff who might have to deal with an outbreak.
3　In the event of rabies becoming established in Britain
(a)　restrictions on the free movement of animals; control of dogs by leash and muzzle; detention of stray dogs and cats,
(b)　control of fox populations,
(c)　compulsory vaccination of dogs with a killed-virus vaccine.
In the absence of rabies in Britain, vaccination of dogs is strongly contra-indicated and the use of attenuated rabies vaccines is illegal. However, if rabies becomes established in the country, vaccination of dogs is the single most effective step in breaking the chain of infection of wild animal→dog→human.

CHAPTER 15

Lassa, Marburg and Ebola Fevers

Three recently recognized viral infections originating in tropical regions of the world have recently come to prominence because of importations to Europe and America. These are collectively referred to as viral haemorrhagic fevers.

Epidemiology
1　Lassa Fever
The virus belongs to the arenavirus group which cause viral

haemorrhagic fever in tropical regions. Lassa fever was first identified in the Lassa Mission Hospital in 1969 and has since been reported from Nigeria, Sierra Leone and Zaire. It is carried by a multimammate rodent from which it spreads to humans. Many of the reported African cases have been mild but on occasion there has been a spread of infection among contacts, particularly in hospitals, causing severe or fatal illness. Since 1969 several severe or fatal cases have been imported into Europe and America, occasionally causing fatal cross-infection among hospital staff. The virus is present in all body fluids and may be excreted in the urine for several weeks after recovery.

2 *Marburg and Ebola virus infections*
A serious outbreak of fever with a substantial mortality occurring in handlers of a consignment of African Green Monkeys to Marburg in Germany led to the discovery of the Marburg virus in 1967. More recently, extensive outbreaks of severe and frequently fatal haemorrhagic fever in Southern Sudan and Zaire were found to be due to a virus, morphologically similar to Marburg but antigenically different from it, which has been named Ebola virus. In Britain, a single case occurred in a laboratory worker handling material from the Sudan outbreak. Marburg and Ebola virus do not belong to any known virus group.

Incubation period

Lassa Fever	7–21 days
Marburg/Ebola Infection	probably shorter

Clinical picture
Lassa Fever. The disease presents with increasing fever, malaise and prostration, persisting for many days. There are few helpful localizing features except exudative tonsillitis which occurs in some severe cases. Other features include conjunctivitis, lymphadenopathy, muscle tenderness and in more severe cases, haemorrhagic manifestations.
Marburg–Ebola Infection. The usual picture is of severe headache, muscle pain and prostration. A maculo-papular rash may be present and many cases have profuse diarrhoea and

vomiting. Haemorrhagic signs develop in the more severe cases which are frequently fatal.

Diagnosis
The most common diseases to be distinguished are malaria, typhoid fever and severe tonsillitis.

Prognosis
In Europeans, Lassa fever has a mortality rate of 50 per cent although amongst Africans larger numbers of milder cases have been reported. Ebola fever has a mortality rate of about 50 per cent and Marburg of about 30 per cent.

Treatment
Concern over the importation of these infections, particularly Lassa fever, has led to the development of elaborate facilities for dealing with suspect cases. When a patient who has been in West Africa within the previous 21 days is reported with undiagnosed fever, the case is first assessed at home by the MOEH and an infectious diseases consultant. If suspicion of Lassa fever remains, the case is removed by special ambulance in which the crew are provided with full protective clothing and microbiological respirators. The suspected case is taken to the nearest high-security isolation unit, usually sited within one of the larger regional infectious diseases departments. These units are self-contained isolation wards equipped with Trexler negative-pressure plastic isolators with adequate back-up facilities of incineration and autoclaves. A restricted list of laboratory specimens, namely blood and faeces for culture (typhoid), blood films (malaria) and throat swabs (tonsillitis), are collected and are examined in secure laboratories. In addition virus swabs, urine and serum are sent by special transport to the Microbiological Research Establishment, Porton, for examination for Lassa, Marburg or Ebola fever, the results being available in seven days. The home is disinfected and quarantined and all first-line contacts, including medical, nursing and ancillary staff are put under daily surveillance when the throat is examined and temperature recorded for 21 days.

For a confirmed case of Lassa, Marburg or Ebola fever, the only treatment at present available is convalescent serum of which a small supply is kept at the London School of Tropical

Medicine; its value is still unproven. Attitudes to the risk of imported viral haemorrhagic fevers have varied from anxiety and panic to the other extreme of ridicule, but in our present state of knowledge, it seems only prudent to handle suspect cases in conditions of secure isolation. Experience has shown that once secure isolation precautions are in operation, the risk of further spread of infection is slight.

CHAPTER 16

Poliomyelitis

Poliomyelitis is an acute infectious disease, caused by a virus which affects the nervous system. The disease presents as a viral meningitis, complicated, in severe cases, by paralysis. In this country, the disease has practically disappeared, as a result of routine vaccination.

Epidemiology
The disease is caused by poliovirus which belongs to the enterovirus group. Poliovirus exists in three antigenically distinct types, termed Types 1, 2 and 3, of which Type 1 is the most virulent. Infection spreads by the faecal–oral route and large numbers of asymptomatic excretors are to be found during an epidemic. Virus is also to be found in the nasopharynx in the acute phase of the disease and may be spread by droplet infection. Factors which predispose to paralysis include physical exertion, pregnancy, tonsillectomy and prophylactic injections.

The epidemiological pattern of poliomyelitis in this country has undergone two major changes in the last 30 years.

Prior to 1947, the disease was uncommon, and paralytic cases were largely confined to very young children, hence the original name of infantile paralysis. It is likely that the virus was very widespread in the community at that time, with universal infection of infants and young children, the former mainly being protected by maternal antibody. The position is still the same in many underdeveloped countries, where standards of hygiene are low, and although there are very few cases of the disease among the local population, visiting Europeans who are unvaccinated suffer a high incidence of paralytic infection.

There was a major change in 1947, when the first of a yearly series of summer epidemics occurred, with 7500 cases and 700 deaths. At about the same time, epidemics were reported from several highly developed countries, notably Scandinavia, Australia and the USA. School children and young adults were most affected and suffered the highest mortality, and the disease tended to occur as frequently in the rural areas as in the towns. It appeared that, as hygienic standards rose in these countries, increasing numbers of people were escaping infection and the subsequent development of immunity, until conditions were ripe for epidemics of the disease. During an epidemic, up to 25 per thousand healthy children were excreting the virus in the faeces, and up to 50 intestinal excretors could be found in association with each clinical case.

A second change began in 1957, with the introduction of vaccines. The earlier killed vaccine was successful in reducing the numbers of paralytic cases, but did not disturb the underlying pattern of virus spread, so that localized epidemics continued among the unvaccinated. In 1962 live attenuated virus vaccine came into use, which not only afforded excellent personal immunity, but prevented subsequent carriage of 'wild' polio virus. In a country where this vaccine is used on a large scale, poliomyelitis is an extremely rare disease, and even the isolation of 'wild' poliovirus from an excretor is a very uncommon event.

Since 1974 following adverse reports on the safety of whooping cough vaccine, the uptake of all other vaccination procedures has fallen to a present national level of just over 50 per cent. Following this inadequate level of protection among children, small outbreaks of paralytic poliomyelitis have occurred in Britain in 1977.

Pathology

The virus enters the body by the intestinal route, and after multiplication in lymphoid tissue there is a short viraemic phase. Virus then settles in the anterior horn cells of the spinal cord and in the cranial nerve nuclei of the brain stem, causing inflammatory changes and, in severe cases, destruction, of these cells.

Incubation period
This is usually 7–14 days, with limits of 3–21 days.

Clinical picture
In some cases there is a short febrile prodromal illness a few days before the main illness develops.

The main illness presents acutely with fever, headache, vomiting and signs of meningeal irritation. In many cases the disease does not progress further and settles in a few days, but in severe cases with neurone damage, flaccid paralysis occurs, with diminished tone and power, and absent reflexes. The paralysis is completely irregular in distribution and extent, and may continue to spread for several days, until the temperature returns to normal. Sensory changes do not occur. The legs and to a lesser degree the arms, are most affected. Paralysis of the bladder with retention of urine commonly accompanies lower limb paralysis, but recovers completely in 2–3 weeks. When the lower brain stem nuclei are involved, bulbar paralysis with weakness of swallowing and coughing develops. This may be an isolated event, with complete recovery in a few weeks, but more commonly is accompanied by extensive spinal paralysis.

Respiratory failure is the most grave complication, and may result from:
1   paralysis of the muscles of respiration,
2   aspiration following bulbar paralysis,
3   a combination of the two.

After the temperature has settled, a slow improvement in paralysed muscles begins, a process which continues for a year or more, but in severe cases is seldom complete.

Diagnosis
The combination of fever, meningeal irritation and flaccid paralysis without sensory changes, is sufficient to establish the diagnosis of poliomyelitis.

The CSF is abnormal, and shows a raised cell count of 50–300 cells which are mostly lymphocytes, although polymorphs may predominate in the first day or so of the illness. The protein is raised to 0·5–1 G/L (50–100 mg per cent) and the sugar level is normal.

Non-paralytic poliomyelitis is indistinguishable from the other types of viral meningitis and leptospirosis, either by clinical or CSF findings.

Paralytic poliomyelitis must be distinguished from acute polyneuritis, particularly acute infective polyneuritis (Guillain–Barré syndrome). In the latter there is symmetrical weakness of the extremities with sensory loss and the CSF shows a normal cell count and sugar level, but a very high protein, often above 3 G/L (300 mg per cent).

Poliovirus can be isolated from the faeces by tissue culture, and paired serum specimens show a rising antibody titre. These results are not available quickly enough to be helpful in early diagnosis.

Prognosis

In epidemic years, the mortality in adults was about 20 per cent, but in children was less than five per cent. Most of the deaths were due to respiratory failure. In severely paralysed cases there is permanent residual disability. In patients maintained by continual artificial respiration, late deaths occur after a period of months or years from repeated and progressive respiratory infection.

Treatment

Paralytic cases are treated in hospital in isolation. The patient is kept completely at rest, with close observation for the development of respiratory or pharyngeal weakness. When the temperature settles and the spread of paralysis ceases, physiotherapy is begun and, at a later stage, orthopaedic aids and surgery may be necessary.

Bulbar paralysis is treated by tracheotomy with the insertion of a cuffed tracheotomy tube. This type of weakness recovers completely.

Respiratory failure due to paralysis of the respiratory muscles alone, or in combination with bulbar weakness, is treated by tracheotomy and artificial respiration. These cases seldom make a useful recovery and are subject to repeated respiratory infections.

Prevention

Cases are isolated for at least 3 weeks, and contacts, especially school children, food handlers or people working with children, are quarantined for three weeks. Minor operations and prophylactic injections are postponed among contacts.

Contacts may be protected by human immunoglobulin (500–1000 mg) but in most circumstances this has been replaced by immunization with live-virus vaccine. The accepted policy is immediate vaccination of all possible neighbourhood contacts with live vaccine. It is therefore very important to notify the Medical Officer of Environmental Health by telephone of the occurrence of a case of poliomyelitis, so that these control measures may be instituted immediately.

Active immunization on a community basis has largely eradicated poliomyelitis. The original Salk vaccine of killed virus gave good individual protection, but has been superseded by the superior Sabin live-virus vaccine. This contains the three strains of virus in an attenuated form, and is administered by mouth in a dose of three drops on a lump of sugar or in syrup simplex. This is recommended for all infants, in three doses, and may be given at the same time as triple vaccine. The vaccine virus colonizes the gut, and produces sound immunity in about a week. A booster dose is advised on school entry. Polio-vaccine virus spreads readily from person to person and with widespread use virtually replaces the 'wild' virus in the community. Until very recently, it was thought that repeated passage of the vaccine virus through the gut did not lead to any increase in virulence. However, most of the recent cases in Britain have been caused by strains intermediate in type between vaccine and 'wild' strains, so that an increase in virulence of vaccine strains is a possibility. Furthermore, in about one case in several million vaccinations, live polio-vaccine causes a major paralytic illness similar to natural poliomyelitis. Several European countries have therefore reconsidered the use of the safer killed-virus vaccine to maintain control of the disease.

Of more immediate importance in this country is the need to re-establish improved uptake of the vaccine among children. The vaccine is not given during any diarrhoeal illness as it is less likely to be effective. It is also contra-indicated in known hypersensitivity to penicillin, streptomycin, polymixin and neomycin, although no serious effects other than transient diarrhoea have been reported when it has been given to penicillin-allergic individuals.

CHAPTER 17

Coxsackie and ECHO Virus Infections

Epidemiology

These are enteroviruses which belong to the picornavirus group. The spread of infection takes place by droplet from the upper respiratory tract of the acute clinical case or, for a longer period, by the faecal-oral route from the faeces of the case or symptomless excretor. Infections have been reported in many countries, and in Britain are most common in the summer months. Cases occur sporadically or in local outbreaks and subclinical infections are common. The highest incidence of clinical illness is in children and young adults. The commonest recognized syndrome is viral meningitis and most of such cases in Britain are caused by these viruses.

A Coxsackie virus infections

These viruses are named after the village in New England where they were first isolated. They are divided into Group A1–24 and Group B1–6. The incubation period is usually 2–5 days, with an upper limit of 2 weeks. The following clinical syndromes occur, but there is considerable overlapping:

1 *Viral meningitis.* This is a benign condition and accounts for half of all diagnosed clinical infections. Rarely a severe encephalitis occurs.

2 *Bornholm disease.* This condition is caused by members of the B group, and has a short incubation period of 2–5 days. The illness starts acutely with fever, malaise and severe muscular pain, usually in a single localized site in the chest or upper

abdomen but may be in the neck or limbs; the diaphragm is most commonly involved. The pain fluctuates in intensity and is greatly aggravated by movement, coughing or deep breathing. In a minority of cases the pain may reappear in a different site after it has settled. Symptoms are usually present for a few days but may last for 1–2 weeks. In family outbreaks the site of the pain will vary in the different members. A relapse a few days after apparent recovery is well recognized. Other manifestations of infection include meningitis, orchitis and pericarditis.

During an epidemic, the disease may be recognized clinically, but it is most unwise to make a diagnosis in the solitary case until many conditions, including pneumonia, pleurisy, appendicitis, cholecystitis, pancreatitis and osteitis, are excluded. There is no mortality.

3 *Simple febrile illness* or undifferentiated upper respiratory tract infection may occur. These may be accompanied by painful inflammatory ulcers in the throat (herpangina), or by inflamed areas with yellow nodular centres in the pharynx (lymphonodular pharyngitis). There may be a maculopapular rash on the trunk and limbs.

4 *Hand-foot-and-mouth disease* comprises a vesicular rash on the extremities associated with vesicles or ulcers in the throat; this is usually caused by Coxsackie A16 virus.

5 *Benign pericarditis* or even severe myocarditis occurs rarely in adults.

6 *Sever disseminated infection*, with myocarditis, hepatitis and encephalitis, occurs rarely in the newborn and may be fatal.

7 *Flaccid paralysis*, similar to paralytic poliomyelitis, occurs very rarely.

B ECHO virus infections

The initials stand for Enteric Cytopathogenic Human Orphan, a name given to this group of viruses before their relationship to clinical syndromes was recognized. Some 34 numbered types are recognized. The incubation period is usually 5–10 days, with limits of 2–14 days. The following syndromes occur, with considerable overlapping:

1 Viral meningitis (most common).
2 Simple febrile illness, often with a discrete macular rash.
3 Undifferentiated upper respiratory tract infection.
4 Outbreaks of gastroenteritis of infancy (rarely).

D

5   Encephalitis, flaccid paralysis or vesicular eruptions in the skin or pharnynx (very rarely).

Diagnosis
Coxsackie and ECHO viruses may be isolated in tissue culture from the throat and faeces and occasionally from the CSF in cases of meningitis. Because of the many virus types, serum antibody tests are only practicable when a particular virus has been isolated and identified.

Treatment
This is entirely symptomatic, with bed rest and analgesics. Encephalitis or generalized infection of the newborn or myocarditis in adults may be fatal, but the other syndromes are benign.

There are no effective preventive measures.

CHAPTER 18

Acute Infections of the Respiratory Tract

In a heavily populated industrial country such as Britain, the most important group of infections as regards prevalence, morbidity and mortality, are those of the respiratory tract. A wide range of micro-organisms may cause respiratory infections, most commonly viruses and bacteria, but occasionally mycoplasma, rickettsiae and chlamydiae. Classification of these infections is difficult, since any one organism is capable of causing differing clinical diseases, and one disease may be caused by a variety of organisms. Viruses, at times, produce characteristic diseases, but at other times they produce simple upper respiratory tract infections without distinctive features. The bacteria may cause primary disease, but more usually they are secondary invaders in a viral infection or where there has been pre-existing lung damage. The two groups of patients who tend to suffer the more serious infections are the very young child and the adult suffering from chronic bronchitis, the 'English Disease'. Table 5 shows the causative organisms and the respiratory disease syndromes associated with them.

TABLE 5

Organism	Specific disease	Comments
1 *Viruses*		
Influenza A	Influenza*	Large scale epidemics
Influenza B & C	Influenza*	Localized epidemics
Parainfluenza	Obstructive	
Types 1, 2 & 3	Laryngitis*	
Respiratory Syncytial	Bronchiolitis of Infancy*	
Measles	Measles	
Adenovirus Types 1–32	Pharyngo-conjunctivitis*	
Enterovirus	Herpangina	Uncommon
Rhinovirus	Common Cold*	
Coronavirus	Common Cold	
2 *Bacteria*		
Strep. pneumoniae	Pneumonia	Primary and secondary infection
Haemophilus influenzae	Acute epiglottitis	Primary
	Pneumonia	Secondary
Staph. aureus	Pneumonia	Primary and secondary infection
Haemolytic streptococcus	Pneumonia	Secondary infection
Klebsiella sp.	Pneumonia	Severe primary—rare
M. tuberculosis	Tuberculosis	
3 *Mycoplasma*		
Mycoplasma pneumoniae	Pneumonitis	Mild illness
4 *Rickettsiae*		
Coxiella burneti	Q Fever (Pneumonitis)	Fatal endocarditis may occur
5 *Chlamydiae*		
Ornithosis Group	Psittacosis (Pneumonitis)	Severe illness
6 *Legionella pneumophila*	Legionnaires disease (Pneumonia)	Severe illness

*Undifferentiated upper respiratory tract infection common.

VIRUS INFECTIONS
Influenza

This is a common highly infectious epidemic disease, characterized by fever and respiratory symptoms.

Epidemiology

Influenza virus belongs to the myxovirus group, and exists in two main forms, A and B. Influenza A is responsible for widespread epidemics or world-wide pandemics of influenza, while Influenza B is associated with localized outbreaks and sporadic cases of influenza, usually of a milder nature.

Influenza A virus has the capacity to develop new antigenic variants at irregular intervals.

The virus contains 2 surface antigens, namely a haemagglutinin or 'H' antigen and a neuraminidase or 'N' antigen as well as a nucleoprotein antigen. The nucleoprotein is fixed but the 'H' and 'N' antigens may change and this is now the basis for classification of the virus variants. Human immunity develops specifically to 'H' and 'N' antigens so that a change in either antigen will result in an almost complete loss of previous immunity. This antigenic shift provides the conditions for a major pandemic of the disease as happened in 1957 and again in 1968. Even a minor antigenic drift in 'H' or 'N' will cause sufficient blunting of immunity to allow a widespread epidemic, as happened in England in 1972. Table 6 shows the major changes which have occurred since the virus was first isolated.

The most serious pandemic of this country occurred in 1918–19 when there were 144000 deaths in Britain and more than 20 million deaths throughout the world. The virus responsible would seem to be identical to the Swine influenza virus, endemic in pigs. Anti-swine haemagglutinin antibodies have been observed in the sera of those born before 1920. In the thirties and early forties, the prevalent virus was Influenza A of the type H0N1 but in 1946 a significant antigenic change occurred and Influenza A1 of the type H1 N1 appeared causing large scale epidemics. This remained the dominant virus until 1957 when another major shift in antigens led to the appearance of Influenza A2 (Asian Influenza) of the type H2 N2, causing a world wide pandemic. There were 10–15 million cases in Britain mainly in young people and there were 5000 deaths, mostly due to secondary pneumonia. There was a low mortality among the

TABLE 6   Influenza A variants

Years of Prevalence	Popular name	Antigenic pattern	Pandemics
1918–19	Swine influenza (Spanish influenza)	A/Hsw$_1$ N1	1918–19
Until 1945	Influenza A	A/HO N1	
1946–56	Influenza A1	A/H1 N1	1946
1957–67	Asian influenza (Influenza A2)	A/H2 N2	1957
1968 onwards	Hong Kong influenza	A/H3 N2	1968
1972 1973 1975 1977	A/England/72 A/Port Chalmers/73 A/Victoria/75 A/Texas/77	Minor antigenic drift of Hong Kong influenza	
1976	A/New Jersey/1976	A/Hsw$_1$ N1	
1977	A/USSR/77 (Red 'flu)	A/H1 N1	

elderly who were found to have serological immunity to this strain, suggesting a similar strain had been prevalent more than 60 years earlier. In the following decade, there were a few smaller outbreaks due to the same virus until 1968 when a new variant emerged known as Hong Kong Influenza of the type H3 N2, which caused a further world wide pandemic. This virus still remains prevalent and seems particularly prone to minor antigenic drift which has lead to successive outbreaks in several parts of the world due to variants A/England/72, A/Port Chalmers/73, A/Victoria/75 and A/Texas/77. It was expected that this variable Hong Kong virus would eventually be replaced by a new strain with totally different surface antigens. However, in 1976 in an influenza epidemic in New Jersey, USA, an Influenza A/New Jersey/76 virus was isolated which had surface antigens similar to the original Swine influenza virus of 1918. This raised fears of a new severe pandemic but so far this has not happened. More recently another virus A/USSR/77 has appeared in many parts of the world including Britain with the H1 N1 antigenic pattern similar to the strain prevalent between 1946 and 1956. The disease predominantly affects persons born after 1957. The reappearance of these older strains lends some weight to the suggestion that there might be a limited number of possible influenza A virus variants.

There is a higher incidence of influenza in the winter months and many epidemics reach a peak in December–January. Infectivity is very high and extends from shortly before the onset of symptoms until shortly after the pyrexia settles. The common occurrence of subclinical infections and the short incubation period both contribute to the very rapid spread of the disease. The mode of transmission is classically by droplet infection, but may be by recently contaminated articles, e.g. handkerchiefs.

Influenza B virus causes sporadic infections and local epidemics about every second year. The disease is usually mild and affects children particularly. It is common in residential schools. In 1973 a new variant of influenza B virus appeared and is now prevalent. This variant also appeared in the Far East and was given the confusing name of influenza B Hong Kong.

The virus may be isolated in tissue culture from throat swabs, gargles, or nasal washings. Immunity after an attack is long lasting and is specific to A and B types as well as to the varying antigens of influenza A.

The highest mortality is usually among the elderly but in the 1918 epidemic, and to a lesser extent in 1957, was relatively high among young adults.

Incubation period
This is usually 1–3 days, with limits of 12 hours to 5 days.

Clinical picture
The illness starts abruptly with fever, shivering and generalized aching in the limbs and back. There is severe headache, aching eyes, soreness and dryness of the throat and a persistent dry cough with retrosternal discomfort. Occasionally there is vomiting or even slight diarrhoea. The fever and symptoms persist for 2–5 days before settling. The cough usually lasts longer, and the patient is often easily tired and depressed in convalescence. Physical examination shows only pyrexia and reddening of the fauces. In epidemics, mild attacks with short-lived fever and less prominent symptoms are very common, possibly due to the presence of some pre-existing immunity.

Complications
1 Respiratory tract
Secondary bacterial infection of the respiratory tract is the most

common complication of influenza and varies in severity from a mild bronchitis to a serious or even fatal pneumonia. Secondary bacterial bronchopneumonia is the most common type occurring one or more days after the onset of symptoms, with gradually increasing cough, purulent sputum and dyspnoea. This is most common in patients with chronic bronchitis. Chest X-ray shows patchy consolidation mostly at the bases. The organisms most often responsible are *Strep. pneumoniae* and *H. influenzae.*

The more rare but very serious variety is fulminating staphylococcal pneumonia which may occur within a few hours or a day of the onset of symptoms. This is seen in young previously healthy adults and presents with the rapid onset of dyspnoea, cyanosis, cough with frothy pink or bloody sputum followed by circulatory failure with icy-cold extremities and absent peripheral pulses. The chest X-ray shows confluent areas of consolidation, the white cell count may show a striking neutropenia and blood culture is usually positive for *Staph. aureus.* Many cases die and post-mortem shows inflammatory and haemorrhagic changes in the lungs from which both *Staph. aureus* and influenza virus may be isolated.

2 Nervous system
Post-infectious encephalomyelitis occurs rarely.

Diagnosis
A clinical diagnosis of influenza is only justifiable during an epidemic, and the labelling of sporadic febrile illness as influenza tends to delay an early diagnosis in many other conditions. The diagnosis may be confirmed by isolation of the virus from the throat, and by a rising antibody titre. The fluorescent-antibody technique is proving to be a satisfactory method of early diagnosis of influenza A. Warning of an epidemic in Britain may be obtained from selected general practitioners acting as 'spotters' and reporting suspected cases to the Public Health Laboratory Service, or from the Department of Health and Social Security weekly sickness returns which tend to rise more rapidly and to a higher level in an influenza outbreak than in any other circumstances. The World Health Organization is responsible for the international surveillance of epidemic influenza and the World Influenza Centre is in London.

Treatment

The uncomplicated case is treated at home in bed with analgesics such as aspirin. Secondary respiratory infection is common in patients with chronic bronchitis, heart disease or renal disease. This complication requires treatment with antibiotics such as ampicillin or cotrimoxazole. Patients with secondary bronchopneumonia are treated in hospital, if possible in isolation, with antibiotics and oxygen. Fulminating staphylococcal/influenzal pneumonia is treated intensively with combinations of antibiotics such as cloxacillin and fucidin, intravenous plasma and large doses of corticosteroids, and oxygen, but the outcome is still often fatal.

Prevention

There are no effective measures for the control of outbreaks although influenza vaccines may play a limited role. In 1957 a killed-virus vaccine from the Asian influenza A (H2/N2) was available and gave 60–70 per cent protection. In 1968 a new saline vaccine from Hong Kong influenza A (H3/N2) and B virus was available and gave short-term protection of 40–60 per cent. Killed vaccines give only short-term immunity. Vaccine is prepared from mixtures of currently isolated influenza A and B strains and so changes in composition from year to year. The current vaccine (1978) contains recently isolated strains of Hong Kong virus and the USSR/77 strain with a current influenza B strain. In addition, a reserve of monovalent A/New Jersey/76 vaccine is held for use in the event of a new pandemic of Swine influenza.

With each change in the virus, a new vaccine has to be prepared and standardized and tends to be in limited supply at the time of the initial large epidemic. Afterwards the vaccines are recommended only for special groups such as chronic heart, lung and kidney disease cases, key hospital and health service staff and residential old people's homes. The vaccine is not recommended for children under 10 years of age, unless significant heart or lung disease is present, when it may be given in a half-dose. Persons allergic to egg are not vaccinated. To maintain protection a single dose is given each year in the autumn. The value of routine vaccination in industry is questionable, particularly since the PHLS trials in Post Office workers have shown no reduction in sick-leave following influenzal vaccination.

The common cold

This is a very common highly-infectious illness, with a mild systemic upset and prominent catarrhal symptoms.

Epidemiology

Although all the respiratory viruses have been identified on occasion, rhinovirus and coronavirus are most consistently isolated from patients with colds. However, in more than half the cases, it is still impossible to detect any virus. Both rhinovirus and coronavirus belong to the picornavirus group, and exist in many antigenically distinct strains. The source of infection is the upper respiratory tract of the case, and the mode of transmission is by droplet infection or close personal contact. Infectivity is high in the early stages of the infection, and spread is facilitated by overcrowding and poor ventilation. On average a person suffers 2 to 3 colds per year, but the incidence lessens with age, presumably as a result of accumulating immunity to the causative virus types. Fatigue or any other cause of lowered resistance may predispose to an attack of the disease.

Incubation period

This is short, varying from 12 hours to 3 days, with an upper limit of 5 days.

Clinical picture

The illness starts with slight pyrexia, tiredness, malaise and irritation of the nasal mucosa and pharynx, with profuse watery nasal discharge, repeated sneezing and coughing. The symptoms subside in a few days, but the nasal discharge becomes thick and mucopurulent, and may persist for a further week. This is the picture seen in adults, but in young children there is usually more pyrexia and less nasal catarrh.

The great majority of colds subside without complication, without treatment and without medical attention. Only symptomatic treatment is necessary in an uncomplicated case. Secondary infection occurs in a minority, causing sinusitis, otitis media or bronchitis. Secondary infection, as expected, is more

D*

common in young children and in adults with chronic bronchitis, and in these cases antibiotic treatment may be necessary.

Prevention

Very little can be done to prevent the spread of colds, and no effective vaccine is available. However, the hardy British habit of ignoring colds undoubtedly results in the unnecessary exposure to infection of vulnerable groups such as babies and chronic bronchitics and public education should be aimed at reducing this risk.

Adenovirus infection

The adenovirus group consists of about 32 serotypes, and is often associated with undifferentiated upper respiratory tract infections. Occasionally a recognizable clinical entity occurs in localized epidemics, comprising fever, conjunctivitis, pharyngitis and lymphadenitis of the neck glands. These epidemics have occurred in school children and industrial workers. The conjunctivitis is the striking feature and is often unilateral. Serotype 8 is particularly associated with keratoconjunctivitis. The disease is more common in the summer. The incubation period is uncertain but may be 5–10 days. There is some evidence that the portal of entry may include the conjunctiva as well as the respiratory tract. Treatment is symptomatic and the disease is self-limiting and benign.

There is some evidence that adenovirus infection may cause mesenteric adenitis, which may mimic acute appendicitis and may be a precipitating cause of acute intussusception in young children.

In infancy, adenovirus is associated occasionally with severe lower respiratory tract infection.

Acute obstructive laryngitis (croup)

Acute laryngitis is an occasional but striking complication of upper respiratory tract infections due to a variety of viruses, the most common of which are measles and the parainfluenza group. There is extension of inflammatory oedema to the vocal cords, epiglottis and pharynx, with considerable narrowing of the airway. There may be associated tracheitis or tracheobronchitis.

Clinical picture

Children under 3 years of age are mostly affected. Shortly after the onset of a simple upper respiratory infection, the voice becomes hoarse, cough assumes a barking quality and there is audible laryngeal stridor. Airway obstruction is common in young children; with recession of the soft tissues of the neck and abdomen on inspiration, and, in the worst cases, cyanosis. The chest is usually otherwise clear on clinical and radiological examination. Fever is not striking and the white cell count is normal or low. In adults and older children, although there is hoarseness, loss of voice, cough and laryngeal stridor, airway obstruction is very rare.

A similar clinical picture may result from acute epiglottitis due to *Haemophilus influenzae* type B. Generally, there is associated septicaemia and the condition is uncommon after the age of seven years. The child is ill and toxic with high fever and severe airway obstruction may occur rapidly. A swollen, angry red epiglottis is characteristic. The white cell count is high. The diagnosis may only be made by laryngoscopy, although an occasional and inconstant clinical sign suggestive of the diagnosis is partial relief of the obstruction by pulling the tongue forward. Diphtheria should always be considered in the differential diagnosis of obstructive laryngitis.

Hospitalization is necessary for most cases, as urgent tracheotomy or endotracheal intubation may be necessary. The child should be nursed in an atmosphere with high humidity. Although most cases are of viral origin, antibiotics should be given in view of the possibility of an *H. influenzae* infection which may be rapidly fatal if left untreated. Chloramphenicol is the drug of choice in acute epiglottitis.

Epidemic bronchiolitis of infancy

Epidemiology

Bronchiolitis occurs, in epidemic form, amongst infants, during the early months of the winter. It is particularly common in the larger towns in the northern half of Britain. It is uncertain whether there has been a substantial increase in this disease, or whether it is now more readily recognized and distinguished from 'bronchopneumonia' of infancy. Recently respiratory syncytial virus has been shown to be responsible for the majority of cases. This disease is seen in its serious obstructive form in young children from 3 months to 3 years of age, more commonly in males. Spread is by droplet infection, often from an older member of the family who is suffering from a simple cold. The mortality is 2–5 per cent in obstructive cases, but the virus may also be responsible for some of the unexpected cot deaths in infancy. Inflammatory oedema and viscid secretion extends deeply into the bronchial tree.

Incubation period
This is not accurately known, but it is probably short.

Clinical picture
About 24 hours after the onset of pyrexia, nasal catarrh and cough, respiratory distress appears. The child becomes pale with a rapid respiratory rate of 40–60 per minute. There is recession of the soft tissues of the neck and abdomen on inspiration, and a longer expiratory wheeze. In severe cases there is cyanosis, which is aggravated by coughing or by attempts at feeding. Most of the severe cyanotic cases are due to the action of the virus itself, but occasionally secondary bacterial infection, often staphylococcal, is responsible. On examination, there are usually showers of fine crepitations over both lungs on inspiration and an expiratory wheeze, but the chest X-ray is often normal or shows only overdistension of the lungs. The obstructive signs persist for several days, after which there is gradual improvement.

Diagnosis
The condition must be distinguished from asthma which is usually recurrent, and from bronchopneumonia where the striking signs of airway obstruction are not normally seen. The virus may often be cultured from a throat swab. In a high proportion of cases, a rapid diagnosis of RSV infection is possible by the immunofluorescent method, preferably from nasopharnyngeal aspirate specimens.

Treatment
Obstructive cases are treated in hospital, in isolation. Severe cases are nursed in oxygen, in a humid atmosphere, and tube feeding is necessary if the infant is distressed by normal feeding. Repeated suction of the pharynx helps to maintain the airway.

Antibiotics have no effect on the viral infection, but are normally used in severe cases where there may be secondary bacterial infection. Corticosteroids in a daily intramuscular dose of 100 mg of hydrocortisone appear to be helpful in some of the severe cases. Tracheotomy does not relieve the airway obstruction but desperate cases, which do not respond to treatment, may be helped by endotracheal intubation with a plastic tube and assisted ventilation.

Prevention

Babies and young children should not unnecessarily be exposed to adults who are suffering from upper respiratory infections.

Vaccine trials were initiated but were stopped by the occurrence of severe clinical reactions (which aggravated the respiratory distress) between serum antibody (including passive antibody transferred from the mother) and virus antigen in the vaccine.

BACTERIAL AND OTHER INFECTIONS

A   Bacterial pneumonias

These are described only briefly in this chapter.

(*i*) *Strep. pneumoniae*

Strep. pneumoniae is the commonest cause of both primary lobar pneumonia and secondary bronchopneumonia.

Pneumococcal lobar pneumonia

This disease is more common in males and during the middle years of life. The source of infection is usually the patient's own upper restiratory tract, but the organism may be transmitted by droplet infection. It is not known why the organism abruptly becomes invasive, but the disease is more common during very cold weather, it is more prevalent during epidemics of influenza and it is common in debilitating conditions such as chronic alcoholism. Infectivity is very slight and case-to-case spread is almost unknown.

Clinical picture. The onset is sudden, with rigors and high fever, pleuritic pain and a cough productive of rusty or bloody sputum. There are physical and radiological signs of consolidation.

Strep. pneumoniae may be cultured from the sputum and the blood culture is also positive in about a third of the cases. Before specific treatment was available, the disease was prolonged and serious with a mortality of about 30 per cent. With penicillin treatment, the temperature returns to normal in 12–24 hours, complications are few and the mortality is very low in previously healthy persons.

(ii) Haemophilus influenzae
This is commonly isolated from the sputum of cases of bronchopneumonia (particularly when this condition is secondary to chronic bronchitis or bronchiectasis) but it is not usually a highly virulent pathogen.

(iii) Staphylococcus aureus
Staphylococcal pneumonia in infancy is a serious disorder usually occurring as a primary infection. The organism is also responsible for many of the more severe cases of pneumonia, secondary to respiratory virus infections.

(iv) Klebsiella sp.
These cause a rare but serious form of lobar pneumonia. The systemic upset is severe and abscess formation in the lung is common. The disease responds slowly to antibiotics such as chloramphenicol and cephaloridine.

(v) Legionnaires' Disease
This disease came to light following an outbreak of severe pneumonia with a substantial mortality at an American legion convention in Philadelphia in 1976. A previously unknown slow-growing Gram-negative bacillus named *Legionella pneumophila* was identified as the cause. Already four antigenically distinct strains of the organism have been isolated. Very little is known as yet about sources of transmission of the infection, although in a recent American outbreak, the organism was found in nearby stream water and also in water present in an air-conditioning system. Since 1976 further cases and outbreaks have been reported from America and Britain. In this country increasing numbers of single cases have been reported and a small outbreak in Nottingham. A number of the cases had recently travelled abroad, particularly in the Mediterranean

area. Outbreaks have been of the 'point-source' type and case-to-case spread appears to be uncommon.

The disease is commonest in middle-aged men, often with a history of heavy smoking and drinking. The illness presents with fever and a marked systemic upset often accompanied by vomiting, diarrhoea and mental confusion. This is quickly followed by increasing cough and dyspnoea with the clinical and X-ray signs of lobar pneumonia. In severe cases an interstitial nephritis and renal failure may occur.

The diagnosis is confirmed by rising antibody titres. In fatal cases the organism may be recognized in lung tissue by immuno-fluorescent techniques.

Erythromycin appears to be the drug of choice so that this antibiotic may be added to the treatment of any severe case of pneumonia on the grounds that Legionnaires' disease may be the cause. Severely-ill cases may require intubation and assisted ventilation. The mortality is 10–20 per cent.

At the present time so little is known about the spread of infection, that there are no recommended preventive measures.

2 Mycoplasma pneumonia

During the Second World War, military personnel suffered a type of mild pneumonia, which did not respond to penicillin treatment and so was named 'primary atypical pneumonia'. An organism was later isolated from the sputum of such cases, which was originally called the 'Eaton agent', but is now identified as *Mycoplasma pneumoniae*. The source of infection is the upper respiratory tract of cases, and spread is by droplet infection. Infectivity is not high and the disease usually occurs sporadically. Occasional outbreaks occur and there was a large outbreak throughout Britain in 1978. The highest incidence is among young adults, and there is no seasonal prevalence. The mortality is negligible.

Clinical picture

Following an incubation period of about 11 days (limits 7–21 days) there is the gradual onset of sore throat, upper respiratory catarrh and fever. A cough develops, which is dry at first but is later productive of mucopurulent or blood-tinged sputum. Patches of crepitations may occur in the chest, but the classical signs of consolidation are rare. Chest X-ray shows one or more areas of consolidation, usually of segimental distribution. The illness lasts 1–2 weeks or even longer, is seldom severe and is usually without complications apart from the rare occurrence of pleural effusion.

The diagnosis is confirmed by a rising mycoplasma antibody titre and rising cold agglutinins in the serum. The organism is difficult to isolate. White cell counts are normal or show a leucopenia.

Treatment

Cases are treated in isolation. The organism is sensitive to tetracycline or erythromycin but the clinical response is not dramatic. The X-ray changes improve only slowly, so that lengthy convalescence is necessary.

There are no effective preventive measures.

3   Q-fever

This rare disease is caused by *Coxiella burneti* which is closely related to the rickettsiae. The infection is endemic in cattle and sheep throughout the world, and is probably transmitted to man by infected dust or milk, although transmission may be by ticks. The disease is most common in animal handlers and outbreaks have occurred from infected milk supplies and among laboratory workers.

The incubation period is 14–28 days, and the onset is abrupt with fever, severe malaise and cough. Severe acute cases show the clinical and radiological features of lobar pneumonia, occasionally with an accompanying hepatitis or other sign of systemic involvement. The diagnosis is confirmed by a rising Phase 2 antibody titre. The treatment of choice is tetracycline, although the response may be slow. Death is very rare in the acute type of infection.

Occasionally the disease presents as a chronic endocarditis which may persist for months or years and may end fatally. The chronic infection responds unreliably to long term antibiotics and surgical valve replacement has been carried out to control the disease with some success. The diagnosis is confirmed by the occurrence and persistence of both Phase 1 and Phase 2 antibodies.

It is possible to isolate the organism, but this procedure is not undertaken routinely because of the risk to staff.

4 Ornithosis

This disease is caused by *C. psittaci* which belongs to sub-group B of the chlamydia group. This group of organisms is intermediate in size and behaviour between rickettsiae and viruses. Sub-group A organisms are responsible for trachoma and lymphogranuloma venereum and there is now a suspicion that some types may be incriminated in non-specific urethritis, a common sexually transmitted disease in Britain.

C. psittaci is distributed throughout the world among birds, which suffer a diarrhoeal illness, the survivors continuing to excrete the organism in the faeces. In Britain, infection occurs in pigeons, poultry and cage birds, such as budgerigars. Spread to man is by handling infected birds or is airborne from dried droppings; case-to-case spread in man occurs rarely. The disease is more severe in the elderly, and occasional outbreaks of severe infection are associated with the unrestricted import of exotic foreign birds such as parrots.

The incubation period is about 10 days, and the onset is sudden with fever, severe malaise, cough and, occasionally, pleuritic pain. Diarrhoea and an erythematous rash are occasional features.There are usually clinical and radiological signs of lobar pneumonia, and in the worst cases there may be hepatic and renal involvement. The diagnosis is confirmed by a rising titre of serum antibody and the organism may be isolated from the sputum or blood.

The organism is most sensitive to tetracycline but the clinical response to treatment is slow. The severe type of infection has a mortality of 20 per cent. The former ban on the importation of foreign birds has now been lifted, perhaps unwisely.

CHAPTER 19

Whooping Cough

Whooping cough is an infectious disease of young children, characterized by paroxysmal coughing, often accompanied by the typical 'whoop', and vomiting. Pulmonary atelectasis is an occasional complication.

Epidemiology

The disease is caused by the organism *Bordetella pertussis*, which may possess 3 surface antigens, termed 1, 2 and 3. The organisms exist in 3 distinct types with the following antigenic patterns 1:2, 1:2:3 and 1:3. Originally type 1:2 was the common epidemic strain but in recent years this has changed to type 1:3. Rarely, a related organism *Bordetella parapertussis* is the cause. The source of infection is the respiratory tract of a case; transmission is by droplet infection, or, occasionally, from recently contaminated articles. Infectivity is high, particularly among close contacts in a household, where few susceptible children escape. Infectivity starts with the onset of catarrhal symptoms, and lasts for up to a month, but does not usually persist for as long as the paroxysmal cough. Abortive attacks occur, particularly in vaccinated children, and are probably the source of a good deal of infection. One attack confers good immunity and second attacks are rare. Infants appear to have very little immunity transmitted from the mother, and the disease is among the more serious infections in the early months of life. Because of the absence of transferred maternal immunity and the difficulty in detecting serum antibody in cases, it is suggested that immunity is mainly of the cell-mediated type.

Whooping cough is endemic throughout the temperate zones of the world, with epidemics occurring at 3- to 4-year intervals each lasting about a year. The most recent epidemic began in September 1977 and in the first 12 months there were about 60000 cases notified and 10 deaths reported. There is no particular seasonal prevalence. The incidence in this country has diminished considerably in the last 18 years, coincident with the increasing use of vaccines. There was a slight increase in prevalence a few years ago which may have been due to the emergence of the previously uncommon type 1:3 organism.

Whooping cough predominantly affects children under the age of seven. Practically all the deaths occur in children under two years of age, and most of these are in babies under six months of age. The fall in mortality, which has been taking place throughout this century, was accelerated by the introduction of antibiotics. Bronchiectasis, once a common result of whooping cough, has largely vanished.

Traditionally, whooping cough is a less severe disease in rural areas than in cities, probably because infection has less opportunity to spread and therefore children are older when they become infected.

Incubation period
This is from 5–14 days.

Clinical picture
The disease begins with low-grade fever, cough and upper respiratory catarrh, which persists for about a week. This is known as the catarrhal phase, and is indistinguishable from many other upper respiratory infections. The fever then settles, but the cough persists and gradually changes in nature, becoming paroxysmal. In a typical paroxysm, the child suffers a succession of prolonged, uncontrollable bouts of forceful coughing. The face becomes congested, the veins stand out and the eyes stream. Sticky mucus is ejected from the nose and mouth during the paroxysm, which terminates with a sudden noisy inspiration called the 'whoop'. The whoop results from a forceful inspiration while the glottis is still partly closed. 'Whooping' may be absent in mild attacks in older children. In infancy, cyanosis is common at the end of a paroxysm. A number of such bouts may follow each other in rapid succession, until the child appears to be distressed and exhausted. Vomiting often occurs at this point. When the paroxysm ends, there is a rapid return to normal composure and appearance; usually there is no coughing between the paroxysms. These paroxysms are repeated throughout the day and become more frequent at night, when they cause a good deal of disturbance both to the patient and to his family. In a case of average severity, the paroxysms vary from 5 to 20 in 24 hours.

It is possible to provoke a paroxysm both by physical and by psychological stimuli. The number and severity of the paroxysms increase gradually during the first week or two, and then gradually decline, the whole process taking from 4 to 6 weeks. When the cough is severe, there may be ulceration of the fraenum of the tongue, subconjunctival haemorrhage, and the expectorated mucus may be blood stained.

Throughout the paroxysmal phase, the temperature remains normal, and abnormal physical signs in the chest are unusual. The child is frequently so well between paroxysms, that it may be difficult for the doctor to reach the correct diagnosis at that time.

Although whooping cough does not relapse, any upper respiratory infection arising during the next few months may cause a temporary return of the whoop.

Complications
These mainly affect the respiratory tract and are more common in babies in poor social circumstances.

(i) *Pulmonary atelectasis*
This is a common complication during the paroxysmal phase, and often cannot be detected by clinical examination. It is due partly to bronchial blockage with viscid mucus, and partly to bronchial and peribronchial inflammation. The extent of the collapse varies from small subsegmental areas to a whole lobe. Any part of the lungs may be affected, but the lower lobes and the right middle lobe are more commonly involved. In most cases, complete re-expansion takes place within 2 or 3 weeks, but in a minority of cases this is delayed for several months. If atelectasis, accompanied by a low-grade infection persists, there is a risk of the development of bronchiectasis; though this has now become rare. Chest X-ray is the only satisfactory way to diagnose and observe the progress in atelectasis.

(ii) *Bronchopneumonia*
This complication is closely associated with atelectasis, and is usually due to secondary bacterial infection. The condition varies widely in severity. Less severe cases may show only a persistent low-grade pyrexia and a slightly increased respiratory rate, without many abnormal physical signs. More severe cases will show a typical bronchopneumonia, with fever, rapid respirations, a tendency to cyanosis, and widespread crepitations and rhonchi.

(iii) *Cyanotic paroxysms*
Cyanosis commonly accompanies paroxysms in babies, and rarely may be followed by a period of pallid apnoea.

(iv) *Convulsions*
Convulsions may occur in whooping cough. These usually

appear to be simple febrile convulsions but when following a cyanotic paroxysm, may be caused by anoxia. Neither type appear to have any lasting sequelae.

Diagnosis
During the early catarrhal phase, the diagnosis can only be suspected from a history of contact.

A persistent paroxysmal cough, worse at night, and accompanied by vomiting, is very suggestive of pertussis. The appearance of the 'whoop' is diagnostic unless there has been a previous recent attack.

Occasionally whooping cough has to be distinguished from:
1   respiratory virus infections (particularly respiratory syncytial or adenovirus);
2   respiratory infections in the course of cystic fibrosis;
3   primary tuberculosis.

The diagnosis can be confirmed in about half the cases, by the isolation of *Bordetella pertussis*, by pernasal swab. Swabs are taken soon after a paroxysm, and should, if possible, be plated immediately on Bordet–Gengou medium. Swabs are more likely to be positive during the first half of the illness, and negative swabs do not disprove the diagnosis.

Differential white cell counts often show a striking lymphocytosis. The total is often in the region of 20000–40000 cells, while the differential count shows 70–80 per cent lymphocytes. These changes are, however, seldom present in infancy.

Complement fixation tests become positive late in the disease but are not usually carried out in routine laboratories.

Prognosis
In recent times, whooping cough has caused the deaths of about 20 children in epidemic years and about 2–4 deaths in interepidemic years. Most of the deaths are in babies under the age of 6 months and are due to bronchopneumonia. So far the present epidemic has caused significantly fewer deaths than previous ones.

Treatment
The older child, without complications, is allowed up and about, and outdoors in good weather. During a paroxysm support and reassurance are needed, and a vomit basin should be near at

hand. Meals are kept small and frequent, and if vomiting is persistent, snacks and drinks are best given soon after a paroxysm. Phenobarbitone is helpful in the case of a highly-strung child, and may reduce the frequency of the paroxysms. Cough mixtures are of no real value. Many treatments have been advocated in the past, ranging from atropine to aeroplane flights, but all are ineffective. Erythromycin and tetracycline are active against *Bordetella pertussis*, and are able to eradicate the organism rapidly from the nasopharynx but tetracycline should be avoided in babies because of its action on teeth and bones; ampicillin is much less active. However, antibiotics do not appear to influence the clinical course of the established disease, except possibly, when given in the early catarrhal stage.

It is important that the child's chest be examined regularly, and a temperature chart kept in order to detect minor respiratory complications. Ideally, every patient should have a chest X-ray towards the end of the illness.

Young babies, and children with definite complications, are best treated in hospital. Babies known to have cyanotic paroxysms require constant nursing observation. During such a paroxysm, secretions are sucked from the pharynx and oxygen is given; if apnoea and pallor develop, mouth-to-mouth artificial respiration is necessary.

Bronchopneumonia requires intensive antibiotic therapy. Combined intramuscular ampicillin and cloxacillin or intramuscular cephaloridine are suitable alternatives for the severe case. Nursing in oxygen is indicated if there is cyanosis, and tube feeding is necessary in infants who are becoming exhausted.

Atelectasis requires prolonged and intensive physiotherapy. Antibiotic treatment with drugs such as oral ampicillin or cotrimoxazole is usually continued until considerable resolution has taken place, even should this require several weeks of treatment. The child is kept under observation until the chest X-ray returns to normal. Convulsions are treated with anticonvulsant drugs such as phenobarbitone, phenytoin or diazepan.

Prevention

The use of whooping cough vaccine appears to have been an important factor in reducing the incidence of whooping cough, although it has failed to eradicate the disease as has virtually happened with diphtheria and poliomyelitis. There is also some evidence that improving social conditions and a falling birth-rate have made a contribution to the lessening incidence and mortality.

In 1974 there was widespread publicity about possible brain damage resulting from whooping cough vaccine and, since that time, only about 30 per cent of British children have received the vaccine. As a side-effect of this controversy, the uptake of the other infancy vaccinations has fallen to an unsatisfactory level of about 50 per cent. While it is accepted that brain damage due to the vaccine may occur in rare instances, the exact incidence is uncertain and it is often difficult to relate the vaccine in a causal way to the brain damage. The present outbreak of whooping cough has occurred in a poorly-vaccinated child population and has been rather larger than the few previous ones, but the disease has been milder.

The Joint Committee on Vaccination of the Department of Health has now strongly advised that routine whooping cough vaccination should continue, but not all responsible medical opinion agrees with this. At the present time national surveys are under way on the side-effects and effectiveness of the vaccine. When the results of these surveys are known and when the full extent and severity of the present epidemic are evident, it should be possible to reassess the value of this procedure in a way that would be accepted by the lay public and the whole medical profession.

The currently-used vaccines contain all the antigenic subtypes including 1 : 3 and booster doses are not advised beyond infancy. Whooping cough vaccine is normally included as a component of 'triple vaccine' in infancy.

The vaccine is not recommended for children with:

(i) a history of convulsions or cerebral irritation in infancy, or with any neurological developmental defect,

(ii) a family history of convulsions or other neurological disorder,

(iii) a current febrile illness particularly of the respiratory tract,

(iv) any severe local or general reaction to a preceding dose.

A personal or family history of 'allergy' is not generally considered as a contraindication.

There is little evidence that vaccine encephalopathy is more prevalent in children with a past history of neurological disease, but rather that the vaccine is inevitably blamed for any subsequent neurological problem.

The protection of the very young baby in a family is a problem which is still not completely solved. The current vaccination schedule means that few babies are vaccinated before the age of the greatest mortality from the disease. For this reason a number of Health Authorities have reverted to a younger age schedule beginning at 3 months and being complete at 6 months of age. Vaccination of the older children in a household reduces the risk of introducing infection but all too often the older vaccinated child develops mild unrecognized disease which is still infectious. Isolation of the baby from other infected children is usually advised but is seldom a successful measure. If whooping cough is introduced into the home by an older child, there is a strong case for giving a 10- to 14-day course of erythromycin to the vulnerable baby as a prophylactic measure, as well as treating the infected child in the same way to eliminate the infection as rapidly as possible.

Exclusion from school of whooping cough contacts is unnecessary.

CHAPTER 20

Streptococcal Infections

The streptococci normally inhabit the upper respiratory and the intestinal tracts.

Classification
A simple but clinically useful classification is based on the type of haemolysis produced on blood-agar plates.

1   Non-haemolytic streptococci e.g. Strep. faecalis
These organisms form part of the normal flora of the gut, and include many anaerobic types. They may cause urinary infections, bacterial endocarditis and intra-abdominal sepsis. They are frequently penicillin resistant.

2   Alpha-haemolytic streptococci e.g. Strep. viridans
These organisms form part of the normal flora of the upper
respiratory tract. *Strep. viridans* readily gains access to the
bloodstream in people with defective teeth and where there is
rheumatic or other types of valvular heart disease the organism
may implant in the damaged valves, causing sub-acute bacterial
endocarditis. It is not intended to describe this disease in detail,
but the usual clinical picture in a patient with valvular heart
disease is of prolonged fever, splenomegaly, progressive anaemia,
multiple sterile emboli and focal nephritis. The disease may be
caused by a variety of upper respiratory or intestinal bacteria,
but *Strep. viridans* is still the most common. The disease
illustrates the great importance of repeated blood cultures in
pyrexial illness. The infecting organism becomes embedded in
vegetations on the heart valve and can only be eradicated by at
least six weeks' treatment with combinations of bactericidal
antibiotics to which the organism is sensitive.

Strep. pneumoniae (pneumococcus) is another member of the
group, and is an important cause of both primary lobar
pneumonia and secondary bronchopneumonia, as well as a
number of less common conditions including meningitis, septicaemia and primary peritonitis in girl children.

3   Beta-haemolytic streptococci
These organisms inhabit the upper respiratory tract.

They were classified by Lancefield into Groups A to G (later
extended). Group A organisms are important human pathogens,
and at one time were referred to as *Strep. pyogenes.* In recent
years, group B haemolytic streptococci have been recognized as
a cause of severe neonatal and puerperal infections. The other
groups are seldom of clinical importance.

A further classification was made by Griffiths into more than
30 Types (since extended). Most of the original Griffiths Types
belong to Lancefield's Group A. Typing is of value in epidemiological investigations. Human immunity to Group A streptococci is Type-specific so that an individual patient may suffer
several infections due to different Types.

Infections due to Group A beta-haemolytic streptococci

The virulence of these infections has diminished in the last few decades, and, as a result, all the clinical manifestations are less common and much less dangerous than formerly.

A wide variety of clinical infections may still be caused by haemolytic streptococci. The particular clinical picture depends on the site of entry of the organism and the production of erythrogenic toxin.

1 Site of entry

(*a*) *The throat and respiratory tract.* Infection results from inhalation of droplets, and the usual 'primary' lesion is a tonsillitis. Occasionally, infection spreads to the surrounding tissues producing the following complications:

(i) Otitis media (via the Eustachian tube). Rarely, mastoiditis, or septic phlebitis of the cranial venous sinuses.

(ii) Paranasal sinusitis.

(iii) Lymphadenitis of the anterior glands of the neck.

(iv) Abscess formation, either retrotonsillar abscess (quinsy) or the more dangerous retropharyngeal abscess.

(v) Rarely, infection of the lower respiratory tract.

(*b*) *The skin.* Infection gains access through a breach in continuity which may be invisible to the eye or may be a wound, burn, leg ulcer or the umbilical stump. In the latter group, local sepsis is usual and this is an important source of cross-infection in hospital.

There is a tendency to spread:

(i) within the layers of the skin, causing erysipelas or impetigo;

(ii) into the deeper tissues, causing cellulitis with occasional abscess formation;

(iii) into the lymphatics, causing spreading lymphangitis and lymphadenitis.

(*c*) *The female genital tract.* Infection gains access only during the puerperium, or following an interrupted pregnancy. Infection may spread from the uterus, causing salpingitis or peritonitis.

(*d*) *Septicaemia.* Rarely, haemolytic streptococci may invade the bloodstream. This is most likely to happen when the primary infection is in the uterus or in the skin (particularly infected burns).

2 Production of erythrogenic toxin

Many haemolytic streptococci (particularly Types 1 to 4) produce an erythrogenic toxin, and, if the patient is susceptible to the toxin, a punctate erythematous rash appears, and the condition is termed scarlet fever. The primary infection is usually in the throat, but may be in a wound (surgical scarlet fever) or in the genital tract (puerperal scarlet fever).

Specific immunity develops to erythrogenic toxin so that usually only one attack of scarlet fever occurs.

Of the many possible varieties of disease which may be produced, only scarlet fever and streptococcal tonsillitis, erysipelas and puerperal infection will be described in detail.

A Scarlet fever and streptococcal tonsillitis

Streptococcal tonsillitis is basically the same disease as scarlet fever, with the addition in the latter of rash and other features due to erythrogenic toxin. Scarlet fever is now the only notifiable streptococcal disease.

Epidemiology

In 1676 Sydenham first differentiated 'scarlatina simplex' from the other exanthemata. Since that time the disease has waxed and waned in severity for no obvious reason. In the mid-nineteenth century, scarlet fever was a severe disease and was a leading cause of death amongst children. At the present time it is a mild condition but is still quite common.

Scarlet fever is found throughout the temperate zones of the world; a seasonal increase occurs during the autumn months. The condition is very uncommon during the first year of life, and reaches its maximum incidence between the ages of 5 and 10 years. The source of infection is normally a case or carrier, and transmission is usually by droplet infection. Infected dust, soiled handkerchiefs and infected articles such as crockery or pencils, may, occasionally, transmit the infection. In the past, several explosive outbreaks due to infected milk or to foods such as ice cream have been reported. In hospitals, infected wounds or burns and, in maternity units, infection of the umbilical stump, have proved to be important sources of cross-infection.

Incubation period

2–5 days.

Clinical picture
The onset of illness is usually abrupt, with fever, headache, vomiting, sore throat and general malaise. The prodromal period, before the rash appears, lasts for 1 or 2 days and during this time signs of tonsillitis appear. The throat shows fiery injection of the tonsils and fauces, and, in more severe cases, flecks of green or white exudate appear on the tonsils. The 'tonsillar' lymph glands in the neck become palpable and tender.

The rash, caused by the erythrogenic toxin, then appears and is described as a punctate erythema. There is a uniform pink blush of the skin, on which many fine red points are visible. This rash first appears on the neck and chest, and spreads downwards to the trunk and limbs in about 24 hours. On the extremities the rash often has a coarser discrete maculopapular appearance. The face is not affected, but there is a characteristic bright flushing of the cheeks with circumoral pallor. The rash persists for a day or two, occasionally for several days. About a week later desquamation occurs in some cases. On the trunk this is of a fine powdery nature, but on the hands and feet it tends to occur later and to consist of larger flakes.

The typical appearance of the tongue in scarlet fever is due to the action of the erythrogenic toxin. For the first 2 days of the illness the tongue is covered with a dense white fur through which occasional red papillae protrude (the white strawberry tongue). About the 3rd day the tongue begins to peel at the sides and tip; by the 4th day it has a red raw appearance with prominent papillae (the red strawberry tongue).

As the rash fades, the temperature settles to normal, and the tonsillar inflammation resolves.

Complications
Otitis media is quite common or a quinsy may develop, but other septic complications such as mastoiditis are now very rare. There are, however, several important 'allergic' sequelae which may develop during the 2nd or 3rd week, and these overshadow, in importance, the original illness.

1   Rheumatic fever
This condition may occur after a haemolytic streptococcal infection and is thought to result from an abnormal antigen–antibody reaction. Any type of Group A streptococcus can

initiate this complication, so the disease tends to recur with reinfection.

The more important clinical maninfestations are:

(a) Fever and 'transient migrating' polyarthritis.

(b) Rheumatic nodules on the extensor surface of the elbows, on the scalp, and over the spine.

(c) Erythema marginatum.

(d) Signs of carditis, namely, tachycardia, continuing during sleep; systolic murmurs, particularly apical; cardiac enlargement; pericardial friction rubs and occasionally effusion; and ECG changes.

The ESR is raised and is usually between 50 and 100 mm/hr; repeat estimations are a useful guide to progress in treatment. The antistreptolysin 0 titre is raised and may be as high as 700 units or more. Rheumatic fever was formerly a common disease, affecting one child in a thousand but has now become very rare. This is presumably due to the reduction in incidence and virulence of streptococcal infections, their ready response to antibiotics and to improvements in nutrition and standards of living.

The age group 5–15 years shows the highest incidence, and poverty and overcrowding appear to be predisposing factors. Recurrent attacks of rheumatic fever, following reinfection with different types of haemolytic streptococci, greatly increase the likelihood of permanent valvular heart disease. To prevent these recurrences, prophylactic penicillin treatment is advised in all cases; in childhood this is continued, ideally, until the age of 20 years, and in adults for a period of 5 years. Suitable preparations are Penicillin V 125–250 mg twice daily, or Penicillin G 200000–400000 units twice daily. Penicillin is normally used in the treatment of an attack of rheumatic fever to eradicate persisting streptococci, along with aspirin or corticosteroids. The latter appear to have some short-term advantage over aspirin in the suppression of symptoms, but have no long-term superiority in preventing chronic valvular heart disease.

2 Acute nephritis

This disease is characterized by:

(a) Fever and oedema of the face and extremities.

(b) Oliguria, with a visibly 'smokey' urine, containing albumen, red and white cells and cellular casts.

(c) Hypertension, occasionally leading to convulsive encephalopathy or to cardiac failure.

About 90 per cent of these cases make a full recovery. The relatively common Type 12 streptococcus is particularly associated with the subsequent occurrence of acute nephritis. In tropical climates, streptococcal skin infections are an important cause of acute nephritis. Since very few types of streptococcus appear to cause nephritis, the condition is not recurrent and prophylactic penicillin is not necessary.

3   Erythema nodosum

This condition is characterized by fever, and the occurrence of raised shiny, tender erythematous areas of various sizes on the lower part of the body, particularly on the shins. As the lesions fade, they exhibit the colour changes of a bruise. There is often polyarthritis and a greatly raised ESR. Although the illness may persist for many weeks, the long-term prognosis is good. It is not specific to streptococcal infection and may occur in primary tuberculosis, sarcoidosis and as a drug reaction, whilst some cases are completely unexplained.

4   Henoch–Schönlein purpura

This childhood condition is characterized by a purpuric rash around the elbows, ankles and over the buttocks, abdominal pain occasionally with diarrhoea and joint pain and swelling. Some cases undoubtedly follow Group A streptococcal infections but, in the majority, the aetiology remains unknown. Gastrointestinal haemorrhage and acute nephritis are recognized complications. Rarely the nephritis becomes chronic but otherwise the cases recover spontaneously.

Diagnosis

The rash must be distinguished from drug or other 'allergic' rashes and even occasionally from measles, rubella and glandular fever. The throat appearance must be differentiated from glandular fever and diphtheria. The throat swab will reveal haemolytic streptococci and white blood cell counts often show an eosinophilia late in the illness.

Prognosis

In the absence of any of the late 'allergic' complications, the prognosis is excellent.

Treatment

Cases are normally treated at home unless complications occur or social circumstances are very unsatisfactory. Bed rest is necessary only until the fever has settled. Penicillin is the drug of choice in all haemolytic streptococcal infections and is usually given for 10 days. Many strains of haemolytic streptococci are resistant to the tetracyclines so that these drugs have no place in treatment. Erythromycin is a satisfactory alternative to penicillin. Throat or nasal carriers of haemolytic streptococci are common and are not usually treated. Occasionally, as in midwives, operating theatre, neonatal or burns unit staff, it is necessary to attempt clearance of the carrier state and repeated or prolonged penicillin is often successful. Local antibiotic creams such as neomycin may help to clear nasal carriage.

The majority of the 'sore throats' seen in general practice are benign short-lived viral infections and antibiotics should be used with discrimination in this type of illness.

Prevention

The patient is isolated at home until the fever and symptoms have completely settled. Children should return to school when complete clinical recovery has taken place; further swab reports and quarantine of contacts are unnecessary. If the patient is returning to a residential school, or to work which carries a particular risk such as nursing, midwifery, food and milk handling, then negative nose and throat swabs should be obtained. For terminal disinfection of the sickroom, 'spring-cleaning' only is required.

An outbreak of streptococcal infection in a hospital ward, school or institution should be dealt with by daily clinical inspection, and by routine swabbing of throat, nose, burns, umbilical stump, etc. Typing of any streptococci found is useful in tracing and containing an outbreak. Prophylactic oral penicillin has been successful in bringing some institutional outbreaks to an end.

B   Erysipelas

An acute febrile illness, associated with an area of tender, spreading cutaneous erythema, which has a well-defined and slightly raised edge.

Epidemiology
Like all haemolytic streptococcal infections, erysipelas has become a less severe illness, in recent years. It may occur in all age groups, but is most common in patients over the age of 40. Chronic disease of the skin, particularly varicose ulceration, is a predisposing factor. Cases occur sporadically and infectivity is very low. The disease tends to recur at intervals in some patients. The organism, which is often carried in the patient's nose, enters through a break in the skin, which may or may not be obvious.

Incubation period
1–7 days.

Clinical picture
The onset is abrupt. There is a short prodromal period with pyrexia, headache, general malaise and often vomiting, lasting about a day, after which the characteristic local erythema appears. This erythema is raised, hot and tender, and has an advancing clearcut edge. The face, and the lower leg, are the more common sites. A 'butterfly' distribution is often seen on the face, with bulbous red swelling of the nose. Facial oedema is common, which may close the eyes and distort the shape of the ears. Superficial yellow blisters, superimposed on the erythema, are common on the face. On the legs or body, a more uniformly smooth area of erythema is seen. In a very severe case, irregular haemorrhagic areas may appear in the erythema. The severity of the illness is proportional to the extent of the erythema.

Complications
Occasionally, erysipelas gives rise to a deeper cellulitis with multiple abscess formation. Following extensive erysipelas of the leg, persistent oedema may occur.

Diagnosis
Facial erysipelas may be distinguished from herpes zoster by the unilateral distribution of the rash in the latter condition. The 'butterfly' rash of disseiminated lupus erythematosis must also be distinguished. Haemolytic streptococci may be isolated from blistering or breaking down areas, and occasionally from the patient's nose or throat.

Prognosis

The mortality of untreated erysipelas was, in the past, in the region of 10 per cent but with modern antibiotic therapy the prognosis has become excellent.

Treatment

Penicillin is the drug of choice. It is given intramuscularly until the pyrexia settles and is continued orally for several more days. Local treatment is unnecessary unless blistering develops when paraffin-gauze dressings may be used. Tetracyclines are not used because of the frequency of resistant strains. In mild cases, oral erythromycin or ampicillin may be used.

Persistent oedema of the leg is helped by elastic stockings.

Prevention

Regularly recurring erysipelas still occurs rarely and long-term penicillin may be used in these cases. The successful treatment of varicose ulceration will remove a commonly predisposing condition.

C Puerperal pelvic infection

This illness is characterized by a rise in temperature, accompanied by local symptoms and signs of pelvic infection in a post-partum woman.

Only a small proportion of pyrexial illness in the puerperium is due to infection in the genital tract; other causes are breast abscess; urinary tract infection; and deep vein thrombophlebitis (leg or pelvic veins).

Epidemiology

'Puerperal fever', due to haemolytic streptococci, was the scourge of maternity institutions in the last century, and was the major factor in the high maternal mortality rate of that period. During the last 50 years, both the incidence and the severity have greatly diminished. Even after a normal confinement, there are raw surfaces and abrasions in the uterus which are liable to become infected. Retained placental tissue provides excellent conditions for the growth of bacteria. Haemolytic streptococci are responsible for some cases of uterine infection but this is now more commonly due to *Staph. aureus*, coliform organisms,

E

non-haemolytic streptococci and anaerobes such as clostridiae and bacteroides sp.

The common sources of haemolytic streptococci in midwifery units are:
(a) The nose or throat of staff or patients,
(b) Instruments or articles infected from the above.
(c) The umbilical stump or skin of newborn infants.

Clinical picture
1   Haemolytic streptococcal infection
There is an incubation period of from one to three days.

The illness starts abruptly with fever, headache, vomiting and general malaise. There are few local pelvic symptoms, and the lochia remains normal in appearance. Occasionally there is rapid spread of infection, causing pelvic peritonitis or even septicaemia.

2   Other infections—'Staph. aureus', coliforms, anaerobes etc.
The onset is often insidious, with low-grade pyrexia, and considerable pain and tenderness in the pelvis. Involution of the uterus is delayed, and the lochia becomes purulent and offensive. Infection may spread to the peritoneum, where it usually remains localized, but occasionally a general peritonitis with paralytic ileus occurs. Rarely a severe septicaemic illness may occur. The more severe cases have a tendency to develop acute oliguric renal failure, particularly in post-abortion sepsis.

Some of the cases have an associated urinary tract infection.

Diagnosis
It is important to exclude infection in other systems particularly the breasts and urinary tract and to examine the calf to exclude deep-vein thrombosis. Pelvic examination is necessary to assess involution of the uterus and tenderness in the pelvis. The cervix is inspected for purulent discharge and a high vaginal swab taken. Other investigations include blood cultures, blood counts and urine examination. All bacteriological specimens should be cultured anaerobically as well as aerobically.

Prognosis
General peritonitis, septicaemia and acute renal failure are all ominous signs, but otherwise the prognosis is excellent.

Treatment
The final choice of antibiotic will depend on the infecting organism and its drug sensitivities. Before this is known, treatment will often be necessary in milder cases with drugs such as oral ampicillin, amoxicillin or cotrimoxazole and in more severe cases with intramuscular cephaloridine or gentamycin. In confirmed bacterioides infections, metronidazole 1–2 g daily is increasingly used. Surgical curettage is delayed until the infection is resolving. The patient is mobilized early to encourage uterine drainage and discourage venous thrombosis.

Prevention
All obstetric procedures require strict asepsis. Staff should be masked, and should not work if they are suffering from an infection of the upper respiratory tract or of the skin. The patient should be isolated at the onset of pyrexia. If a haemolytic streptococcus is found, a thorough investigation must be carried out among the staff, patients and babies, in order to discover and to remove the source of infection. Typing of streptococci is essential in such an investigation.

CHAPTER 21

Staphylococcal Infections

Epidemiology
Two main types of staphylococci are differentiated by their cultural appearance and coagulase reaction. *Staph. albus* which is coagulase negative is a very minor pathogen, occasionally responsible for superficial sepsis. Coagulase-positive *Staph. aureus* is at times a dangerous human pathogen. Many types pf *Staph. aureus* may be differentiated by phage typing.

Staph. aureus frequently colonizes the nasopharynx and the skin, particularly the axillae and perineum, without causing disease. The organism can survive outside the body for long periods, in dust and blankets, an important factor in hospital cross-infection.

Clinical picture

Staph. aureus is capable of causing a wide variety of human
diseases, mostly of a suppurative type.

1   Infections of the skin and subcutaneous tissues

Staph. aureus is the cause of septic spots, boils, carbuncles,
furunculosis of the ear, sycosis barbae, impetigo and the bulk of
wound sepsis and superinfection of burns. These are usually
localized superficial infections, requiring only local treatment.

Impetigo. The relative roles of streptococci and staphylococci
in the aetiology of impetigo remain uncertain. Mixed infections
are frequently found and it appears that either organism may be
the primary invader. In the tropics, pure streptococcal impetigo
is common and is an important cause of acute nephritis. The
initial lesions in impetigo are vesicular which coalesce and break
down rapidly to yellow-brown crusts. The lesions may occur
anywhere on the body but are most common around the nose
and mouth. The scalp may be involved in patients with
pediculosis.

Toxic epidermal necrolysis. In the related but less common
condition, toxic epidermal necrolysis (sometimes called
Ritter's disease) *Staph. aureus* of phage type 71 has been
consistently isolated from the skin lesions in children. The
disease presents with pyrexia and widespread erythema over the
body with impetiginous crusting round the eyes, lips and skin
folds of the neck. Superficial blistering then occurs in the
erythematous areas. These lax serum-filled blisters rupture within 24 hours and the superficial layer of skin strips away like
wet tissue paper leaving a raw red surface which dries and heals
in a few days. Most cases run a benign course but occasionally
there is considerable loss of serum from the blistered areas with
falling blood pressure. In infancy the condition was formerly
known as pemphigus neonatorum and is more severe with an
increased risk of generalized infection. In adults a similar
clinical syndrome occurs; this is not usually staphylococcal in
origin and is more commonly a drug reaction.

In infancy, colonization with *Staph. aureus* takes place within
a few days of birth, and septic spots, infected umbilical stump
and 'sticky eye' are common. These infections must be taken
seriously, because of the ease with which generalized infection
can develop and because of the risk of spread of infection in baby

nurseries. Breast abscess in the mother is liable to follow infection in the baby.

In adults, boils and carbuncles of the nose and upper lip are potentially dangerous, because of possible spread of infection via the facial veins to the cranial venous sinuses resulting in a serious septic thrombophlebitis. In some patients boils occur in successive crops which persist for long periods. In these cases there is often heavy colonization of the carrier sites, nose, axillae and perineum. Persistent boils tend to occur in diabetes, so the urine should be tested for sugar.

2 Infections of the respiratory tract

Staphylococcal pneumonia is most common in babies and elderly people, particularly those debilitated by some other disease. It may follow respiratory viral infections such as measles or respiratory syncytial virus infection but the most severe fulminating and frequently fatal form complicates epidemic influenza in young adults. One or several lobes may be involved. Soap bubble cysts (pneumatocoeles) in chilfren and abscess formation in adults are characteristic features.

Staph. aureus is the predominant primary respiratory pathogen in children with cystic fibrosis, although in cases on long-term chemotherapy, this tends to be replaced by pseudomonas and proteus species.

3 Infections of the gastrointestinal tract

(*a*) *Staphylococcal enterotoxin food poisoning.* Staph. aureus can multiply in certain foodstuffs, and elaborate a heat-resistant toxin, which, on ingestion, causes an acute gastroenteritis.

Epidemiology. Food is usually infected by a handler who is a nasal carrier of staphylococci or who has an infectious skin lesion; occasionally milk becomes infected when a cow is suffering from staphylococcal mastitis. If infected food is left at room temperature for several hours, the organisms multiply and produce the enterotoxin. Even if the food is subsequently cooked so that the staphylococci are killed, the enterotoxin will withstand boiling for up to one hour and the disease may still occur. The whole process is more rapid in hot weather and most outbreaks occur in the summer. Prepared meats, pies and cream cakes are commonly responsible. The disease usually appears in sudden outbreaks, and single cases are not easily recognized.

Incubation period. This is very short, averaging from two to four hours, with limits of from one to six hours.

Clinical picture. The onset is abrupt with abdominal discomfort, intense nausea and repeated vomiting. The patient is pallid and feels dizzy and faint. The loss of gastric acid may cause a transient alkalosis with tetany and muscle cramps, while the loss of fluid occasionally results in dehydration. Diarrhoea occurs after a few hours but is usually not severe or persistent. The patient recovers rapidly after about 24–48 hours.

Diagnosis. The sudden occurrence of acute vomiting, particularly when it occurs in a number of people simultaneously, together with epidemiological evidence of a very short incubation period, suggests the diagnosis. When the foodstuff has not been heat-treated since the original infection, the isolation of staphylococci from it, and from the vomit and faeces of patients, confirms the diagnosis and phage typing is useful in establishing the relationship of organisms isolated. Tests for the identification of enterotoxin are available in many centres.

Treatment. Most cases recover quickly with a period of bed rest, and adequate fluid intake. Severe cases, where alkalosis or dehydration is present, may require intravenous saline. In spite of the dramatic symptoms, there is virtually no mortality.

Prevention. This depends on the observance of high standards of hygiene by food handlers, and the exclusion from work of those with septic skin lesions. The use of automated procedures in the preparation, wrapping and transport of food, and the use of refrigeration in storage are valuable preventive measures.

(*b*) *Staphylococcal enterocolitis.* Overgrowth of staphylococci in the bowel following antibiotic treatment may produce a severe enterocolitis, mainly affecting the ileum. This condition is rare and has recently been differentiated from the commoner pseudomembranous colitis which occurs in similar circumstances but is due to a toxic clostridial superinfection. Both conditions are common in middle-aged or elderly patients who have undergone abdominal surgery and who have been treated with antibiotics. The finding of *Staph. aureus* in faeces specimens in hospital patients is a common event and does not in itself justify a diagnosis of enterocolitis.

4 Infections of the urinary tract
These include perinephric abscess and chronic pyelonephritis.

5   *Infections of bone and joints*
These include acute osteitis and septic arthritis, both of which may lead to chronic suppurative disease.

6   *Generalized infection*
This is an uncommon but serious manifestation of staphylococcal infection. The initial septicaemia often follows a localized infection, such as a boil, septic skin lesion or infected burn. The disease may be fulminating and rapidly fatal, with sustained high fever, tachycardia, and a tendency to peripheral circulatory failure. In these cases there is profound toxaemia with signs of cerebral irritation, shown by altered consciousness or coma, together with gastrointestinal irritation shown by vomiting and diarrhoea. The disease may take a more leisurely course, with less fever and toxaemia, but with the development of metastatic abscesses in the lungs, kidneys, heart valves, brain or bone. These metastases will eventually dominate the clinical picture. In patients who survive the acute stage of a fulminating staphylococcal infection, there is a tendency for acute anuric renal failure to develop.

7   *Hospital infections*
Staph. aureus with its widespread distribution, robustness and tendency to develop antibiotic resistance, has been one of the most successful organisms to flourish in the hospital environment. Originally the organism was sensitive to all antibiotics, but slowly increasing percentages of resistant organisms have replaced the sensitive strains, particularly in hospitals. At present, most hospital strains are resistant to penicillin, about half to streptomycin and the tetracyclines and a small percentage to chloramphenicol and erythromycin. Surgical and maternity units are most at risk. Many of the outbreaks of infection have been caused by organisms of a few phage types, such as Type 80. At the present time, with the development of such drugs as cloxacillin, fucidin and cephaloridine, many of the tragic results of hospital cross-infection can be averted, but already resistant strains to the newer drugs are beginning to emerge, so the respite may be short-lived.

In hospital the following factors combine to aggravate the problems of staphylococcal cross-infection.
1   The high incidence of antibiotic-resistant organisms.

2   A high carrier rate among hospital staff, with a correspondingly high count of the organism in dust and blankets.
3   The introduction of 'open' cases of staphylococcal disease.
4   The congregation of a population of debilitated people,
subject to surgical operations, radiotherapy, intravenous procedures and treatment with cortisone and cytotoxic drugs, all of
which increase susceptibility to infection.
5   The congregation of newborn babies in maternity units.

The control of staphylococcal disease in hospital depends on
the more discriminate use of antibiotics, the isolation of cases of
'open' infection and the better control of infection in the
environment, with particular reference to dust and blankets.

Treatment
Most of the benign local forms of skin infection require only
simple local treatment. Abscess formation requires surgical
treatment, and antibiotic therapy is no substitute for this.

Patients with 'open' staphylococcal disease should be isolated.

Antibiotics
For local superficial infections, such as impetigo and septic
spots, local antibiotic preparations are available. The drugs used
tend to be those which are not used systemically, and include
neomycin and bacitracin. In patients suffering from recurrent
boils, local treatment may not arrest the tendency to crop. In
such cases better results may result from daily baths, followed
by dusting of the axillae and perineum with a talcum powder
containing 0·5 per cent hexachlorophane (sterzac) and treatment
of the nose with neomycin and hibitane ointment (Naseptin).

In severe cases of impetigo, and in all cases of toxic epidermal
necrolysis, full doses of a systemic antibiotic such as cloxacillin
or erythromycin are given, in addition to local treatment.

In more serious systemic staphylococcal infection, systemic
antibiotic treatment is necessary. In some conditions, such as
breast abscess, perinephric abscess and empyema, surgical drainage is the essential treatment, and antibiotic treatment by itself
may disguise or prolong the illness. In other conditions, such as
pulmonary and septicaemic infections, antibiotics play the main
role in treatment. In yet other conditions, such as osteitis and

brain abscess, antibiotic treatment, given early, may sterilize and cure the infection, but in delayed cases, surgical drainage may become necessary.

It is essential to determine the antibiotic sensitivities of the staphylococcus rapidly, as this is the most important guide to the choice of drugs. At the present time the production of new antibiotics has outstripped the large-scale development of drug resistance and this offers a choice from a number of satisfactory drugs. Penicillin is still the drug of choice, when the organism is known to be fully sensitive but when treatment has to start before the sensitivity is known, an antibiotic effective against penicillin-resistant strains must be chosen. There are several effective alternatives:

1   Cloxacillin may be given orally or intramuscularly depending on the severity of the infection, in divided doses totalling 2–4 g per day. The newer derivative flucloxacillin is much better absorbed after oral administration and has largely replaced oral cloxacillin.

2   Erythromycin is useful for infections of the skin and subcutaneous tissues particularly in patients allergic to penicillin. It is given orally in daily doses of 2 g.

3   Fucidin (fusidic acid) is a powerful synthetic antibiotic which is very useful in the treatment of a variety of severe staphylococcal infections. It penetrates deep tissues readily and retains activity in the presence of pus. It is particularly useful in bone and joint infection, and is given orally in a dose of 1–2 g daily. In severe infections it can be given intravenously. There are few toxic side-effects. It does not share cross-resistance with other antibiotics but resistance to the drug can develop quickly during treatment. This may be avoided by using fucidin in combination with another drug such as erythromycin.

4   Lincomycin is another useful antistaphylococcal drug and can be given either orally or intramuscularly. It penetrates bone readily and is of value in treatment of both acute and chronic osteomyelitis. A derivative, clindamycin, is many times more powerful and is also available in a parenteral form, so is replacing lincomycin. However, both these drugs have been implicated in pseudomembranous colitis.

5   Cephalosporin derivatives such as cephaloridine are highly effective against penicillin-resistant staphylococci. Cephaloridine is a bactericidal drug and is also active against a wide range of

E*

Gram-positive and Gram-negative infections, and so is particularly useful in many severe respiratory infections including those due to staphylococci and Klebsiella species. It is not absorbed from the gut and so is given by intramuscular injection in doses of 250–1000 mg 6 hourly. For less severe infections cephalexin is an absorbable oral preparation of the same group with the same range of activity. The daily dosage is 1–4 g. Patients allergic to penicillin may also be allergic to these drugs.

6   Finally, gentamicin, a bactericidal aminoglycoside antibiotic, is highly active against both Gram-negative infections and *Staph. aureus*. The drug is ototoxic and nephrotoxic and as the margin between therapeutic and toxic levels is small, the dosage is monitored by peak and trough blood levels. The dosage is about 80 mg three times daily by intramuscular injection.

In severe infections, particularly when septicaemia is present or suspected, it is wise to choose a combination of two bactericidal drugs from cloxacillin, fucidin, cephaloridine or gentamicin. Profound toxaemia and peripheral circulatory failure are frequently present in such cases and supportive treatment with intravenous plasma and large doses of corticosteroids may gain valuable time until antibiotic treatment begins to be effective.

In staphylococcal enterocolitis, the essential part of treatment is adequate replacement of lost fluid by intravenous drip. The antibiotic already in use is immediately withdrawn and may be replaced by a narrow spectrum oral antibiotic such as cloxacillin or erythromycin, when the staphylococcal aetiology is established.

CHAPTER 22

Diphtheria

Diphtheria is caused by infection with virulent strains of *Corynebacterium diphtheriae*, and is characterized by membrane formation in the throat, and by the absorption of an exotoxin which damages heart muscle and nervous tissue.

Diphtheria is now very rare in Britain as a result of over 30 years of routine immunization.

Epidemiology

There are three types of *C. diphtheriae*, namely gravis, intermedius and mitis. The source of infection is the throat or nose of a case or carrier, and transmission is usually by droplet infection. When cases are occurring, the carrier state is common, but is usually temporary. The disease is most common in children and very mild attacks can occur among the immunized. In several recent local epidemics, the infection has been imported from abroad, as diphtheria is still endemic in many parts of the world. In England and Wales prior to 1940 there were each year on average 55000 cases and 3000 deaths. The introduction of community immunization in 1940 resulted in a rapid decline in the incidence. In the last 12 years there have been only 116 cases with 12 deaths (averaging 10 cases per year with 1 death), mostly of the mitis type. In the last few years the uptake of immunization has fallen nationally to little more than 50 per cent and this has increased the likelihood of outbreaks of the disease.

Pathology

The causative organism settles in the superficial debris of the tonsils, where some toxin is produced, which causes necrosis of the epithelium and results in membrane formation. In the membrane, the organism continues to multiply with the production of larger amounts of toxin which, after being absorbed into the bloodstream, becomes fixed in heart muscle and nerve tissue. Toxin is readily absorbed from the fauces but only slightly, if at all, from the nose, larynx or skin.

Incubation period

This is short, varying from 2–5 days.

Clinical picture

The disease presents with sore throat, pyrexia, general malaise, headache and vomiting. The sore throat is not severe and may not be mentioned by a child. The membrane first appears on one or both tonsils, but may spread onto the pharyngeal wall, the palate or the buccal mucosa. The membrane persists and may spread for several days and then gradually separates and disappears, leaving a reddened mucosa. In gravis infections the membrane tends to be thin and greyish, and is likely to be associated with marked cervical adenitis and periadenitis which results in the classical 'bull neck' in the most severe and gravely toxic cases. Occasionally petechial haemorrhages in the skin and bleeding from mucous membranes accompany a highly toxic infection. In mitis infections, the membrane is usually thick and creamy and readily spreads to the pharynx and larynx. Laryngeal diphtheria may occur without faucial involvement but more commonly results from spread of the membrane from the throat. In the larynx, the membrane is likely to cause airway obstruction with the development of hoarseness, croupy cough and laryngeal stridor. Later and more serious signs are inspiratory recession of the soft tissues of the neck and abdomen, profuse sweating, pallor or cyanosis.

When the primary infection is in the nose, there is likely to be a bloodstained nasal discharge, which is usually unilateral. In tropical countries, diphtheritic infection of cutaneous ulcers or sores occurs and this may be the source of an imported outbreak.

Complications

These result from the effect of toxin on heart and nerve tissue. The toxin becomes fixed in tissues during the first few days of the illness, and cannot afterwards be neutralized by antitoxin.

Heart

Toxic myocarditis, with hypotension and a variety of cardiac arrhythmias, occurs between the 10th and 20th day. If this complication is not fatal, complete recovery ensues.

Nervous system

Toxic neuritis occurs from the 3rd to 7th week. The palate is most commonly involved, causing nasal speech and regurgitation of fluids. The pupil reactions and eye movements are next most commonly affected. More rarely, bulbar paralysis, or the involvement of the spinal nerves, may occur, and may lead to respiratory failure. All paralyses recover completely, in time.

Diagnosis
Diphtheria has to be distinguished from anginose glandular fever, tonsillitis, quinsy, agranulocytosis and blood dyscrasias. The laryngeal form must be distinguished from the other causes of laryngeal obstruction. *C. diphtheriae* is isolated by throat and nasal swabs, but treatment should not be delayed whilst awaiting the result, if the circumstances are highly suspicious.

Prognosis
Mortality is 5–10 per cent and depends on the degree of toxicity of the infecting organism, the pre-existence of immunity in the patient, and the stage at which treatment is commenced. The causes of death are grave toxaemia (haemorrhagic signs often signify a fatal outcome), or laryngeal obstruction in the early days; heart failure during the 2nd or 3rd week, or respiratory failure at about the 6th week.

Treatment
Antitoxin remains the standard treatment of diphtheria. Given on the 1st day, antitoxin reduces the mortality to nil, but when delayed until the 4th day, the death rate is about the same as in the untreated disease. Dosage varies from 8000 to 80000 units depending on the severity of the illness. Up to 20000 units are given intramuscularly in a single dose, but where larger doses are required, the intravenous route is also used. Reactions are less common with the modern refined antitoxin, but, as the preparation contains horse protein, the following manifestations may still occur:
1   Immediate anaphylaxis, with pallor, dyspnoea, collapse and hypotension, which can be rapidly fatal. This type of reaction is most likely to occur in patients who have previously received horse serum in some form, or who give a history of allergy, such as hay fever or asthma. These two groups of patients should be given a test dose and should be observed for signs of a general reaction for a period of about an hour before the main dose is given. The test dose for the group who have previously had horse serum is 0·2 ml of antitoxin, and for the 'allergic' group is 0·02 ml followed in an hour, if no reaction develops, by 0·2 ml. Anaphylaxis is treated by intramuscular adrenaline, and by hydrocortisone intravenously.

2   Delayed serum reactions occur after about 10 days, with fever, rash, and joint pain with swelling.

After treatment with antitoxin, there is normally no further spread of the membrane. The patient is kept at rest until the risk of cardiac complications is past, and remains under observation throughout the period when late neurological complications may occur. Erythromycin is the most effective antibiotic and is given in a 10- to 14-day course.

Where there is laryngeal involvement, the aim of treatment is to preserve the airway, and tracheostomy may be necessary.

Symptomless persons with positive throat or nose swabs are commonly discovered in association with cases and are now usually isolated in hospital. Healthy carriers with a recorded history of previous immunization are treated with a 10- to 14-day course of erythromycin and are given a booster dose of formal toxoid. Infected susceptible contacts are treated with a dose of 1000–2000 units of antitoxin in addition to erythromycin, active immunization being carried out later. Both cases and carriers are isolated until 3 successive nose and throat swabs at 2-day intervals are negative. Further nose and throat swabs are taken at home at weekly and later, monthly intervals for a period of 4–6 months to detect late reversion.

Prevention

The virtual eradication of diphtheria is the result of a national compaign of active immunization commencing in 1940. Immunization is available to all infants in the first year of life, as part of the routine vaccination programme. A booster dose is given at school entry, combined with tetanus toxoid. This regime gives virtually complete protection. The recent drop in the level of immunization in children, resulting from the controversy over whooping cough vaccination, is a cause for concern and efforts need to be made to improve this situation.

Further immunization is unnecessary in the general population, although it is known that immunity levels drop gradually and that up to a third of adults will lose measurable immunity. A problem does arise in maintaining immunity in adult health service staff such as medical, nursing, ambulance and laboratory staff who may come into contact with the disease or older children and adults who are close contacts in a diphtheria outbreak. Routine immunization with normal vaccine (containing 25 Lf doses) is not acceptable over the age of 10 years because of the higher incidence of severe local reactions. A low-dose diphtheria vaccine (containing 1·5 Lf doses, combined with tetanus toxoid) may be used and provides an effective boost of immunity in over 95 per cent of adults, without significant ill-effects (combined adsorbed diphtheria and tetanus toxoid for adult use). Following the use of this vaccine, the Schick test may be used to confirm immunity. Otherwise Schick test and control is carried out in all cases to avoid the vaccination of immune patients (Schick negative) or allergic patients (Schick toxin and control positive).

Schick test—0·2 ml of a diphtheria toxin preparation is in-jected intradermally and the site is inspected after 1–3 days. In a non-immune person there is an unopposed inflammatory re-action due to the toxin, showing as a red indurated area at the injection site. In an immune person, antibody neutralizes the toxin and no reaction is seen. False-positive reactions occur in some persons who are both immune and allergic; these are detected by the simultaneous use of a control injection in the other arm (the same preparation but with the toxin neutralized by heat). The true positive (non-immune patient) will have a red reaction at the toxin site but not at the control site. The false-positive (immune and allergic patient) will have a similar red reaction at both sites, and does not require further vaccination.

The control of a local epidemic requires thorough and repeated searches for cases and carriers among household contacts, neighbours and school contacts, by throat inspection and by nasal and throat swabbing, and the isolation of all positive persons. When a school is involved in an outbreak, medical inspection and swabbing are greatly facilitated by keeping the school open, although all children reported absent are immediately visited. In primary schools, the entire school is swabbed but in secondary schools, this is usually not necessary.

Corynebacterium ulcerans infection

Rarely from a case of sore throat, the related organism *C. ulcerans* is isolated. This organism is probably of animal origin but can produce mild toxic diphtheria with membrane for-mation in the throat. The case requires the standard manage-ment of diphtheria, but as the infection does not spread beyond the immediate family, wider control measures are unnecessary.

CHAPTER 23

Infections of the Gastrointestinal Tract

In the less developed regions of the world, infections of the gastrointestinal tract cause a high morbidity and mortality. These infections may be caused by worms, flukes Protozoa, bacteria and occasionally viruses, and the problems are aggravated by low standards of sanitation and hygiene, malnutrition and inadequate medical services. In developed countries such as Britain, bacterial and non-specific intestinal infections are common although the mortality is low. In the case of immigrants and travellers returning to Britain, unusual conditions such as amoebiasis or cholera need to be investigated, and if hospital admission is necessary, the case should be in strict isolation.

Acute diarrhoea is a common problem in international travellers. Apart from recognized intestinal pathogens, several other factors including changes in diet and climate and alteration of the usual faecal flora may contribute to the aetiology of 'travellers' diarrhoea'. In a few recent outbreaks, unusual strains of *Escherichia coli* have been incriminated.

Many of the intestinal infections have features in common:
1 They are acquired by ingestion of water or food, either contaminated directly by the infected excreta of man or animals, or indirectly by hands or articles infected from the same faecal sources.
2 Diarrhoea is a feature common to many of the infections.
3 Symptomless carriers or excretors are common sources of infection.
4 The diseases tend to occur in outbreaks, often of a point-source type.

Several important preventive measures have reduced the incidence of these diseases in developed countries:
1 Provision of pure water supplies.
2 Provision of safe sanitary disposal of excreta.

TABLE 7

	Organism	Disease	Comments
1	PROTOZOA		
	Entamoeba histolytica	Amoebiasis	Chronic diarrhoea is usual. Hepatic abscess is common.
	Giardia lamblia	Lambliasis	Chronic diarrhoea in infancy. Acute diarrhoea in travellers.
2	BACTERIA		
	Salmonella typhi	Typhoid fever	
	Salmonella paratyphi A, B and C	Paratyphoid fever	'Gastroenteritis' and symptomless excretors are common alternatives.
	S. typhimurium many other types	Gastroenteritis (food poisoning)	Rarely causes severe septicaemic disease.
	Shigella sonnei, *Sh. flexneri* and *Sh. dysentery* and *Sh. boydii*	Dysentery	Mild illness in Britain.
	Specific types of *E. coli*	Gastroenteritis of infancy. Travellers' diarrhoea	*E. coli* only appears to account for a small minority of cases.
	Vibrio cholerae	Cholera	El Tor variety recently replaced classical strains.
	Vibrio parahaemo-lyticus	Gastroenteritis (food poisoning)	Infection from raw seafood, particularly crab meat.
	Campylobacter sp.	Gastroenteritis	Animal sources common.
	Staph. aureus	1 Enterocolitis 2 Gastroenteritis due to toxin (food poisoning)	'Hospital' disease.
	Clostridium perfringens (welchii)	Mild gastroenteritis (food poisoning)	Particularly affects the elderly.
	Clostridium botulinum	Botulism	Very rare.
	Bacillus cereus	Gastroenteritis	From recooked rice
3	VIRUSES		
	Enterovirus	Mild gastroenteritis	Uncommon
	Rotavirus	Gastroenteritis of infancy	Common in winter.

3 Hygienic standards in preparing and protecting food supplies.

4 Control of known human carriers, who are not permitted to engage in work involving the handling of food.

5 Refrigeration of food.

These diseases are now classified by their causative organisms, the more important types being listed in Table 7. The older term 'food poisoning' is still used and refers to sharp outbreaks of illness affecting a number of persons, occurring within a short time of a shared meal. In the prebacteriological era, food poisoning was thought to be a single clinical entity but it is now recognized as covering several different infections which fall into two main types:

(i) *Toxin type.* The illness is caused by the ingestion of preformed toxin produced by bacteria present in contaminated food. An example is staphylococcal food poisoning (incubation period 1–6 hours).

(ii) *Bacterial type.* The illness is caused by the ingestion of living bacteria in contaminated food. An example is salmonella infection (incubation period, commonly 12–24 hours).

CHAPTER 24

Typhoid and Paratyphoid Fevers

These diseases are caused by a group of invasive members of the salmonella group, and are characterized by a bacteraemic illness with prolonged fever and with relatively inconspicuous gastrointestinal symptoms.

Epidemiology

Typhoid is caused by *Salmonella typhi*, and paratyphoid by *Salmonella paratyphi* A, B and C.

Typhoid fever

Salmonella typhi is a purely human pathogen so that the source of infection is the faeces or urine of a human case or carrier. The disease is usually acquired by ingestion of contaminated food or water. In Britain in the past, outbreaks were usually water-borne but in recent times have mostly been food-borne. The incidence in Britain has dropped steadily in the present century due to the provision of safe water supplies, safe sewerage disposal and improved food trade practices. At the present time, some 200–300 cases occur each year. The majority of these are adults and acquire the infection abroad, most commonly from the Indian subcontinent, occasionally from Mediterranean countries or elsewhere. About 10 per cent of the cases have not been outside Britain, although some of these (mainly children) are associated with a chronic carrier originally infected abroad. Direct case-to-case spread is uncommon, occurring in less than 10 per cent of incidents.

An infected contact may occasionally remain a symptomless excretor but usually clinical illness occurs. Infectivity lasts throughout the clinical illness and often for several months afterwards during the period of convalescent carriage. One per cent of cases become permanent carriers. Faecal carriers are the most common, the infection often persisting in the bowel and biliary system. Urinary carriers are rare but present a particular risk.

Any age group may be affected but the highest incidence of disease is in the young adult. Babies seldom acquire the disease, but when they do so it tends to take a mild and atypical form. Lasting immunity follows an attack of typhoid.

A number of strains may be identified by phage-typing and this is useful in the investigation of cases and outbreaks.

Paratyphoid fever

Paratyphoid B is the most common type and most cases are imported from abroad. The organisms occur in both man and animals and so the epidemiology is more similar to intestinal salmonellosis. Outbreaks are usually food-borne and the organism may require a period of multiplication in a suitable food-stuff in order to produce the necessary high infecting dose. Symptomless carriers are common during outbreaks.

Convalescent faecal carriage is common but usually clears within a few months.

Pathology
Early in the illness the organism becomes established in the bloodstream and is widely disseminated particularly to the reticulo-endothelial system. There is probably a secondary invasion of the bowel via the liver and biliary tract. The Peyer's patches are then involved and in severe cases may ulcerate. After the acute illness, low-grade infection may persist indefinitely in the bowel, biliary tract, kidney and bone.

Incubation period
This is usually 7–14 days, with limits of 3–21 days. For paratyphoid, it lies normally towards the shorter limit of the figures given.

Clinical picture
The onset of typhoid is usually insidious, with headache, malaise and abdominal discomfort. The patient may remain ambulant for much of the 1st week. During this week the temperature mounts gradually, eventually reaching a consistently high level, although the pulse, by comparison, is slow. Constipation is usual, and there may be slight abdominal distension. A persistent cough is common and epistaxis may occur.

During the 2nd week, the temperature remains high, the abdominal discomfort may become more marked, and diarrhoea develops in half the number of cases. The patient is weak and listless and is now usually bedridden. Facial pallor contrasts markedly with the flushed appearance noticed in many other febrile conditions. The spleen usually becomes palpable and an erythematous rash, described as 'rose spots', appears on about the 10th day in more than half the cases. The rash consists of small macules, usually on the abdomen, flanks or chest. It erupts in several crops each lasting only a day or two. It is sparse, often with no more than a dozen lesions at one time and may not be visible on a pigmented skin. In some cases, signs of bronchitis or bronchopneumonia appear.

During the 3rd week, the fever remains high. In a severe attack the patient may become extremely weak, muttering and delirious with abdominal distension, a condition formerly called the 'typhoid state'. The highest incidence of gastrointestinal complications occurs during the 3rd week.

During the 4th week, the temperature gradually returns to normal, and the symptoms and abdominal distension subside, although the patient is listless and anorexic for some time afterwards.

In untreated typhoid, about 10 per cent of cases suffer a relapse 1–3 weeks after the apparent termination of the illness. The relapse is usually of milder and shorter duration than the initial illness.

The clinical picture of paratyphoid is often similar to the above, but the illness is usually milder and less protracted although the rash may be more profuse. A common alternative presentation of paratyphoid, particularly in children, is that of an acute gastroenteritis, in which the diarrhoea is very marked, but the fever and systemic upset are less.

Complications

These have become rare with the advent of specific chemotherapy.

1   Gastrointestinal tract

(*a*) *The 'typhoid state'* was formerly thought to be the result of 'toxaemia' but is now known to be, to a large extent, the result of severe electrolyte disturbance and, particularly, to the loss of potassium.

(*b*) *Haemorrhage* is most common during the 3rd week when sloughs in the intestinal ulcers separate. Bleeding varies from streaks of blood in the stool, to a severe haemorrhage with the passage of copious melaena or of bright red blood, when sudden faintness, thirst and the signs of shock are superimposed upon the already present typhoid symptoms.

(*c*) *Perforation* of an ulcer in the ileum is also most common during the 3rd week; this accident usually presents with sudden severe abdominal pain and rigidity of the abdominal wall, followed by increasing abdominal distension. Pain is not always present, and perforation should be considered whenever there is sudden deterioration in the condition of a patient; an X-ray of the abdomen in the upright position may show air under the diaphragm.

(*d*) *Cholecystitis* is common, but is usually subclinical, and is an important factor in subsequent faecal carriage.

2   Osteitis
This is very rare, and occurs, silently, during convalescence usually in rib, vertebra or tibia. The lesion is chronic and may break down months or years afterwards, the discharge from the sinus being infectious.

3   Other complications
These include the following:
(a) Myocarditis with peripheral circulatory failure.
(b) Pyelonephritis which may persist as a low grade infection associated with long-term urinary carriage.
(c) Deep-vein thrombosis in the legs.

Diagnosis
A clinical diagnosis may be possible, particularly in a patient returning from abroad but the following investigations are always necessary:
1   Blood culture, is positive during the first two weeks, and occasionally later. It again becomes positive during a relapse.
2   Faeces and urine culture may be positive at any time in the illness, particularly during the 2nd and 3rd weeks.
3   White cell counts show a leucopenia, with a neutropenia.
4   The Widal test measures the agglutinins which appear in the blood during the disease. There are two separate types in both typhoid and paratyphoid, the 'H' (flagellar) and the 'O' (somatic), and a 3rd type only in typhoid, the 'Vi' (mouse virulence) agglutinin. In enteric fever, agglutinins usually appear during the 2nd week, with a steep rise in 'H' titre and a smaller but more significant rise in 'O' titre, which reach a peak during the ensuing weeks and fall gradually over a period of months or years. The peak 'H' and 'O' titres are so variable that diagnostic levels cannot be quoted and in a minority of cases no antibody appears in the blood. The interpretation of raised antibody titres must take into account the current clinical and bacteriological findings, a previous history suggestive of typhoid or other salmonella infection and previous TAB vaccination. The 'Vi' agglutinin usually appears in low titre during the later stages of the illness, and its persistence for a prolonged period,

even in a titre of 1:10, is suggestive of the carrier state. Persistent low 'H' and 'O' titres may follow TAB vaccination or an attack of typhoid and may undergo a non-specific rise in any new febrile illness, a possible cause of confusion.

Prognosis

Formerly, the mortality of untreated typhoid was over 10 per cent, and of paratyphoid about two per cent, but specfic therapy has reduced these figures to less than one per cent.

Treatment

(*a*) *The clinical disease*

Cases are treated in isolation, in hospital. Chloramphenicol is the drug of choice in a daily dose of 2 g for an adult and 50 mg/kg for a child. With treatment, the temperature returns to normal in about 4 days, the symptoms abate, and the risk of complications is largely removed. Chloramphenicol is continued for 4–5 days after the temperature becomes normal. Relapses respond quickly to a further short course of chloramphenicol. Although the organisms are usually sensitive *in vitro* to a number of antibiotics, none has proved to be as consistently effective as chloramphenicol. However, outbreaks of chloramphenicol-resistant typhoid have recently occurred in Mexico and Vietnam and in these cases cotrimoxazole or amoxicillin may have to be used. Severe cases, including those in the 'typhoid state', require full biochemical assessment and urgent replacement of any deficiencies which may be revealed, particularly those of potassium and sodium chloride. Corticosteroids were formerly recommended in severe typhoid, but there is little real evidence to support their use.

Intestinal haemorrhage is treated with blood transfusion. Intestinal perforation is treated surgically if the patient's general condition is satisfactory, but otherwise, conservatively by gastric suction, intravenous fluid and supplementary antibiotics.

(*b*) *The carrier state*

Convalescent carriage is common, but clears spontaneously in most cases and does not require antibiotic treatment. Chronic carriage represents a difficult therapeutic problem. Chloramphenicol does not affect the carrier state, and the other antibiotic regimes which have been advocated (including ampicillin 3 g daily for three months or cotrimoxazole in a month's course), usually fail to eradicate the infection. Cholecystectomy is only recommended when X-ray examination shows clear cut evidence of gall-bladder disease. Persistent carriers are a long-term public health problem.

Prevention

1 The most important measures are:

(a) the provision of pure water supplies,

(b) the safe sanitary disposal of excreta and

(c) high standards in the handling, processing and storage of foodstuffs.

2 TAB vaccine provides a substantial if incomplete protection against typhoid and it is of doubtful value in paratyphoid. Monovalent antityphoid vaccine is claimed to cause fewer reactions than TAB but is only now generally available. Two doses of vaccine at 4–6 weeks interval, a further dose in one year and booster doses every three years are necessary to maintain protection. Local and general pyrexial side-effects are common with this vaccine.

Vaccination is recommended for the following groups:

(a) Members of the Armed Forces (given as combined TAB and tetanus vaccine, usually by intradermal injection).

(b) Family contacts of chronic carriers.

(c) Persons travelling abroad, except to North America and Northern Europe.

The vaccination of hospital staff is not now considered to be necessary.

3 Typhoid cases in hospital require six consecutive culture-negative specimens of faeces and urine before they are discharged. Further specimens are examined at regular intervals for several months, as excretion may be intermittent, and blood is examined for 'Vi' antibody over the same period.

4 During an outbreak a search is made for the source of infection, including missed cases, symptomless excretors, carriers and the examination of suspect water supplies, foodstuffs and sewage. Phage-typing of organisms may be helpful in tracing the infection.

5 Known chronic carriers are kept under observation by the Medical Officer for Environmental Health. Carriers who observe

careful personal hygiene are safe in the community, but are not allowed to work in a food trade, under the *Public Health (Infectious Diseases) Regulations 1968.*

CHAPTER 25

Salmonellosis

The salmonellae are a large group of intestinal pathogens, present in many animal species. They frequently cause acute diarrhoeal disease in man, often from the ingestion of contaminated foodstuffs.

Epidemiology
Over 1000 types of salmonellae are recognized throughout the world, and about 200 have been found in Britain. Two thirds of all human salmonella infections are due to a single type, *S. typhimurium*. Other common types isolated in recent years are *S. agona, S. enteritidis, S. hadar, S. heidelberg, S. ibadan, S. indiana, S. newport, S. panama, S. stanley* and *S. virchow.*
    The following sources of infection are important:
1   Human cases with diarrhoea are highly infectious, and many excrete the organism for weeks or months afterwards. During an outbreak, excretors without clinical disease are common.
2   Domestic species, notably cattle, pigs and poultry, commonly have intestinal or bacteraemic disease, so that abattoirs and butchers' shops may become heavily contaminated, and meat, chicken and all products are sources of infection. Infected imported animal foodstuffs and fertilizers contribute to this source.
3   All domestic pets may be intestinal excretors. Fresh pet foods are commonly contaminated and may be a source either via infection of the pet or by being stored along with human food.

4 Duck eggs are a well-known source of infection, the organism being present inside the egg. Hens' eggs also may convey infection, but only from the outside of the shell.

5 Frozen poultry inadequately thawed before cooking is a common source of infection.

6 Rats and mice are frequent excretors, and may directly contaminate exposed food or may transmit infection to other domestic animals.

There has been an increased incidence of salmonellosis in the last 30 years. Spread of infection has been encouraged in animals by intensive or 'battery' farming methods using bulk-imported foodstuffs and in humans by an increase in communal feeding. Including school children, about half the population eat one meal per day away from home. In more than half the cases reported, infection has been conveyed by processed meat dishes such as pies, inadequately cooked sausages, stews, and reheated preparations. Other foods commonly involved are cream, cake fillings, trifles and custards, none of which are heat-treated prior to consumption. Contaminated food is in no way altered in appearance, taste or smell. The bacteria often require a period of multiplication in the foodstuff, in order to reach a dose capable of causing disease, and this is more likely to occur in the warmer summer months. Most reported episodes involve single cases, but an entire family may be involved, and occasionally more widespread outbreaks occur.

The exact mechanism of diarrhoea production is not clearly understood but probably involves fluid and electrolyte transfer defects in the small bowel and mucosal inflammation in the large bowel.

Incubation period
This is usually 12–24 hours, with limits of 6–72 hours.

Clinical picture
The onset is abrupt with vomiting, watery diarrhoea which may contain blood and mucus, abdominal discomfort and colicky pain. There is usually pyrexia, headache and malaise. Loss of fluid may cause thirst, pallor, dizziness and lassitude. Physical examination shows only some diffuse abdominal tenderness. The pyrexia and symptoms may persist for several days or occasionally longer before gradually settling. Cases may continue

to excrete salmonellae in the faeces for weeks or months after the illness.

Complications
Dehydration
Severe diarrhoea leading to dehydration is particularly liable to occur in the very young, in the elderly and in those with reduced gastric acidity from previous gastric surgery or atrophic gastritis. Hypotension and shock leading to acute renal failure may occur in such cases.

Invasion of the bloodstream
Occasionally, salmonellae may invade the bloodstream causing a more severe illness with high protracted fever and a marked systemic upset. Septicaemia may lead to metastatic infection in the meninges, lungs, bones or joints. Sometimes, the resulting illness may resemble typhoid or paratyphoid fever with little or no diarrhoea and in recent years, *S. virchow* from infected poultry has been responsible for a number of such cases.

Colitis
Salmonella infection may occasionally cause a severe colitis with profuse bloody diarrhoea which may be difficult to distinguish from ulcerative colitis or Crohn's disease. Rarely, toxic dilatation of the colon may occur.

Diagnosis
In the individual case, the diagnosis is confirmed by the isolation of the organism from the faeces. Blood culture is essential in severe cases. Sigmoidoscopy, rectal biopsy and barium X-rays may all be necessary to distinguish salmonella colitis from ulcerative colitis or Crohn's disease. In an outbreak, rapid investigation of suspected cases, carriers, animal sources, food remains, and food preparation premises, is carried out. Phage-typing is a valuable measure in tracing infections.

Prognosis
The mortality is 0·25 per cent of notified cases. Most deaths are due to septicaemia or dehydration and renal failure, and occur in the elderly or the very young, often in patients who are already suffering from some pre-existing disease.

Treatment

Uncomplicated cases are treated at home with bed rest and an adequate fluid intake, including electrolyte supplements if the diarrhoea is severe or protracted. Antibiotics are contra-indicated in cases of enteritis as they do not influence the course of the disease, either clinically or bacteriologically. Septicaemic cases do require antibiotic treatment and chloramphenicol is the drug of choice, although ampicillin and cotrimoxazole are possible alternatives. Dehydrated adult cases require intra-venous fluid, initially normal saline or Darrow's solution (potassium-containing fluids are avoided if renal failure is suspected).

Antibiotics are of no value in the treatment of persistent carriers and in fact there is evidence that they may prolong the carrier state.

Prevention

High standards of hygiene are essential in all food premises such as shops, factories, slaughterhouses, kitchens and restaurants and all are periodically inspected by Environmental Health staff. Food is protected from animals, rodents, insects and dust. Raw and cooked meats should be handled and stored separately. Food should be cooked or thoroughly reheated before use whenever possible and frozen food should be completely thawed before cooking. Food should be stored in refrigeration.

Any food handler who develops diarrhoea should be excluded from work until proved clear of infection. Known salmonella carriers are excluded from all food-handling until cleared. Carriers may return to other types of work or to school, after instruction in personal hygiene; it is particularly important to wash the hands after going to the toilet.

CHAPTER 26

Dysentery

Dysentery describes a group of infections characterized by enterocolitis with diarrhoea often containing blood. The two main types are amoebic dysentery of the tropics and the less protracted bacillary dysentery which occurs throughout the world.

1 Amoebic dysentery

This is a common and frequently serious disease occurring widely throughout Asia, Africa, the Middle East and South and Central America. The disease is caused by the protozoal organism *Entamoeba histolytica*. It spreads by the faecal–oral route usually through the agency of infected food or drinking water. In active intestinal disease, the organism is in the motile amoeboid form which invades the bowel wall. A non-motile cyst form of the organism is present in the bowel of a substantial percentage of the population of endemic areas; this form is not necessarily associated with active disease but contributes to the spread of infections. In most cases the infection is confined to the intestinal tract but in a minority it spreads via the portal circulation causing hepatitis or liver abscess. Amoebiasis is occasionally found in travellers returning to Britain but rarely spreads in this country.

Intestinal amoebiasis. This presents with diarrhoea, often containing traces of blood and mucus and accompanied by intestinal colic, malaise and variable pyrexia. These symptoms may persist or recur over a period of weeks or even months. In severe cases the diarrhoea consists largely of blood and mucus and the systemic upset is marked. The diagnosis is confirmed by the finding of motile amoebae in fresh faeces specimens examined immediately under the microscope. The organism is most abundant in the mucus. Sigmoidoscopy is useful for obtaining a diagnostic faeces specimen but the appearance of the mucosa is similar to that seen in other inflammatory conditions such as ulcerative colitis. A serum antibody test is positive in rather more than half the cases.

Hepatic amoebiasis. This may occur with or without a preceding dysenteric illness and takes the form of localized hepatitis or of liver abscess. The illness presents with sustained pyrexia, a severe systemic upset and occasional upper abdominal pain. The liver may be enlarged and tender but jaundice is unusual. Amoebae are seldom found in the faeces, but the serum antibody test is positive in most cases. The presence of a liver abscess may be demonstrated by radioactive liver scan. A chemotherapeutic trial may be justified if the diagnosis remains in doubt.

Treatment. Metronidazole is the drug of choice in both forms of the disease. In intestinal infections it is given in a dosage of 800 mg three times daily for a week and in hepatic disease 400 mg three times daily for the same period. Liver abscess will usually resolve slowly with one or more courses of metronidazole and surgical drainage is usually unnecessary. In a minority of cases a relapse may occur necessitating retreatment. In Britain, cyst excretors may be treated with metronidazole to prevent reactivation of the disease but with uncertain results.

Older treatments such as emetine and chloroquine were less effective and more toxic and so are now seldom used.

2 Bacillary dysentery

The causative organisms are the Shigella group, which consists of four main types, *Shigella sonnei, Sh. flexneri, Sh. dysenteriae* and *Sh. boydii.* In this country most of the cases are caused by *Sh. sonnei,* with a minority caused by *Sh. flexneri.* A number of strains of *Sh. sonnei* may be differentiated by colicine typing but this is only of value in the study of epidemics. The source of infection is the faeces of a case or carrier, and the infection usually spreads directly from case to case, particularly where personal hygiene is lacking. The disease is most common in young children, and is particularly troublesome in residential children's homes. Adults are sometimes infected by contact with children in families, schools or hospitals. The period of infectivity is from the time of infection until the organism disappears from the faeces, although the case with diarrhoea is much more highly infectious than the carrier with formed stools.

The carrier state does not usually persist for more than a few weeks, and long-term carriage is very rare. An attack of the disease appears to confer immunity. The disease is endemic throughout the year with an increased incidence in the winter months, and is commoner in urban areas. About 20000 cases are notified each year in Britain.

In tropical countries dysentery is more often caused by *Sh. dysenteriae* or *Sh. boydii* and tends to be a severe and protracted disease. It is often food-borne or spread by flies.

Incubation period
This is usually 2–4 days, with limits of 1–7 days.

Clinical picture
The onset is usually abrupt, with a short period of headache, malaise, fever, anorexia and abdominal discomfort, soon followed by diffuse lower abdominal colicky pain and diarrhoea. Vomiting is common at the onset, but is not persistent. Diarrhoea may continue for a week or longer, and in severe cases contains blood and mucus.

Mild cases with slight malaise and looseness of the stools for a day or two are very common, and many infected cases remain entirely asymptomatic, although excreting the organism.

In young children, febrile convulsions sometimes occur at the onset. In some cases there is an associated upper respiratory tract infection.

Diagnosis
Dysentery may be clinically indistinguishable from the other infectious diarrhoeas, and the diagnosis is established by the isolation of shigella organisms from faeces specimens or rectal swabs.

In the baby, intussusception must be kept in mind while in the young adult other causes of bloody diarrhoea such as ulcerative colitis and Crohn's disease must be considered. In the older patient, ischaemic colitis, diverticulitis and carcinoma come into the differential diagnosis. Sigmoidoscopy with biopsy and barium enema may be necessary.

Prognosis
Bacillary dysentery in Britain is usually a benign disease. The

1–2 deaths reported each year are usually associated with pre-existing disease in young infants or the elderly.

Treatment

In the majority of cases, the only management necessary is bed rest and fluid replacement while the symptoms persist. In the average case there is little to be gained by the use of antibiotics but in the occasional severe case, possibly of tropical origin, a course of ampicillin or cotrimoxazole may be worthwhile. In the comparatively rare protracted carrier state when the patient is unable to return to work the same antibiotics may be used. Since many strains are resistant to a range of antibacterial drugs, it is necessary to obtain antibiotic sensitivities before such use. The type of antibiotic resistance found tends to spread to other coliform organisms in the environment by the transfer of plasmid carrying resistance factors.

Prevention

Important preventive measures are the provision and proper use of toilets, washing facilities and clean towels in schools and institutions. In an outbreak disposable paper towels should be used and the regular disinfection of toilets (seat, chain and doorhandles) should be carried out. Although the value of home isolation is doubtful, in a residential institution the immediate isolation of a child who develops diarrhoea may prevent an outbreak. The usual policy is to allow cases to return to school or work after they have completely recovered clinically, without further faeces culture. However, cases or carriers engaged in food-handling trades are not permitted to return to work until repeated faeces cultures are negative. This has legal backing under the Public Health (Infectious Diseases) Regulations 1968, although a carrier excluded under these regulations is entitled to financial compensation.

There is no need to exclude close contacts from school or work, except in the case of food-handlers who are better excluded until faeces cultures are known to be negative.

CHAPTER 27

Gastroenteritis of Infancy

Gastroenteritis is a common infectious disease in infancy characterized by vomiting and diarrhoea and associated with a variety of bacterial and viral causes. Salmonella and shigella infections are excluded from consideration because of differing epidemiological and clinical features. Although gastroenteritis can occur at any age, it is more prevalent and more prone to complications in the first two years of life and so is essentially a disease of infancy. The most important complication is dehydration.

Epidemiology
In many cases of gastroenteritis, no causative agent is found, but several aetiological factors are established:
1 The disease is rare in exclusively breast-fed infants, who have a lactobacillary faecal flora which resists colonization with coliform organisms.
2 Since 1973, rotaviruses (so-called because of a wheel-like appearance) have been demonstrated by electronmicroscopy in the faeces of about 30 per cent of cases of gastroenteritis and the existing evidence suggests that rotaviruses are a significant cause of infantile gastroenteritis throughout the world. The viruses are closely related to animal viral pathogens causing diarrhoea in calves and in infant mice. In Britain, rotaviruses are most frequently found in the winter months and may account for the increased incidence of gastroenteritis in the winter.

The role of other viruses remains uncertain. In a few outbreaks, enteroviruses or adenoviruses have been isolated but these do not seem to play a significant role in the aetiology. Recently, coronaviruses which are important causes of enteritis in pigs and calves, have also been demonstrated by electronmicroscopy in the faeces of some gastroenteritis cases but a causal role has not been established.
3 Toxigenic strains of *E. coli* probably account for up to 20 per cent of cases. The organisms elaborate an enterotoxin

similar to cholera enterotoxin and the diarrhoea is produced by the toxic effect on the fluid and electrolyte transport mechanism of the small bowel mucosa, without any visible inflammatory response. These toxigenic strains are generally identified by the possession of specific 'O' antigens and are agglutinated by the corresponding antisera. A large number of such strains are recognized, the more important being 018, 026, 044, 055, 086, 0111, 0114, 0119, 0125, 0126, 0127, 0128 and 0142. It is becoming apparent, however, that not all agglutinable strains are toxigenic and conversely some toxigenic strains are nonagglutinable. Toxin production is an irregular feature, so that the virulence of any strain varies greatly. It is possible to demonstrate toxin production experimentally but this is not yet a routine test.

4   The infectivity of gastroenteritis, whether or not it is associated with agglutinable *E. coli* or viruses, is both variable and unpredictable. Children over the age of two years are rarely affected in an outbreak.

Although there is no demonstrable aetiology in many cases of gastroenteritis, a possible hypothesis is that the condition may be a temporary upset in intestinal function resulting from the colonization of the infant gut with a new strain of coliform organism. In this context the agglutinable *E. coli* strains may cause disease by their colonization effect as much as by being pathogenic bacteria. This hypothesis is in accord with the immunity of breast-fed infants who resist coliform colonization and also the relative immunity of children over two years of age who would have already met the majority of new colonizing strains. The same hypothesis might also explain the common condition of 'traveller's diarrhoea', which is seldom caused by the specific pathogenic organisms, but has been shown on occasion to be associated with agglutinable *E. coli*. The diarrhoea occurring with antibiotic therapy may be similarly due to an imbalance in the normal bowel flora.

In the early part of this century, gastroenteritis appeared in large summer epidemics, and was a common cause of death. In developing countries, the disease is still one of the major factors in infant mortality. During the last 50 years, the death rate in Britain has fallen steadily from around 50 to less than 1 death per 1000 births; nevertheless the disease remains a major problem of child health in this country. The disease is estimated to affect about 10 per cent of babies per year and is commoner in the industrial North than in the South of England. The disease is most common in the 2–4 months age group, and has a higher incidence in the winter months in Britain, whereas in the poorer countries it is predominantly a summer disease. The mode of spread is probably by contamination of feeds and feeding utensils from faecal sources, and, because overcrowding and low standards of hygiene predispose to the transference of infection, the disease is commoner in the poorer industrial areas.

Infectivity is very variable but tends to be higher in baby nurseries and hospitals, where premature or debilitated infants are particularly at risk. After an attack, the infant appears to have some immunity, but may remain infectious for a considerable period. Some infants suffer several attacks of the disease before the age of two years. From time to time, epidemics of severe gastroenteritis have occurred, usually in children's hospitals. The clinical course has been more severe and prolonged, the infectivity greater and the mortality higher. These outbreaks have been associated with one of the specific *E. coli* types.

Incubation period
The incubation period is speculative, but where case-to-case spread has been observed in institutions, the incubation period has been less than 12 days.

Clinical picture
The severity of the disease is very variable. The mildly affected infant is disinclined to take feeds and has looseness of the stools for a day or two before he returns to normal health. In the more severe case, vomiting after feeds is usually the first symptom. The infant often refuses further feeds, and looks pale and irritable. Diarrhoea starts about 24 hours later and usually becomes the predominant feature. Pyrexia is variable. The severity of the diarrhoea varies from 3 to 4 loose stools daily, to hourly watery stools which contain little or no faecal material. When severe diarrhoea persists, electrolyte disturbance and dehydration are liable to occur. On examination, the infant is usually pale, there may be slight abdominal distension, and some cases may show signs of respiratory tract infection. The illness persists for a period varying from 1 to 2 days to a week

or more, before recovery begins. Severe cases may occasionally suffer one or more relapses.

In the rare hospital epidemic type of disease, the onset is insidious but the diarrhoea becomes severe and persistent or relapsing. There is progressive weight loss and there may be repeated episodes of dehydration. In the later stages there may be jaundice and hepatomegaly, with a tendency to gastrointestinal haemorrhage. Death usually occurs after a wasting illness lasting several weeks.

Complications

Dehydration

Dehydration is the most important complication and clinical grading is useful, as it correlates fairly well with the degree of weight loss.

Grade 1 dehydration (*mild*). The infant is crying, irritable and sleepless. Haemoconcentration results in pallor of the skin with contrasting bright redness of the lips. The eyes are slightly sunken. This appearance represents $2\frac{1}{2}$–5 per cent loss of body weight.

Grade 2 dehydration (*moderate to severe*). The infant is irritable or apathetic and has a striking appearance. The face is pallid and pinched and the eyes are deeply sunken with prominent black rings below them. The skull and facial bones become more prominent. The conjunctiva is dry and reddened. The anterior fontanelle is sunken and the mouth is dry and sticky. The skin loses elasticity and this may be demonstrated by the persistence of a pinched-up fold of skin or by the fine wrinkling which occurs when a broad fold of skin is compressed between finger and thumb. Urinary output is scanty. This appearance represents 5–10 per cent loss of body weight. The facial appearance and the skin signs of dehydration may be considerably obscured in obese infants.

Grade 3 dehydration (*severe with peripheral circulatory failure*). This is an extremely dangerous condition. In addition to marked signs of dehydration, the infant is limp and apathetic and the skin is grey and mottled. The extremities are icy cold and the peripheral pulses are not palpable. This appearance represents 10–15 per cent loss of body weight.

Acidosis is a common feature of dehydration and results in

rapid gasping respiration which is readily mistaken for respiratory tract infection, particularly in fat babies in whom the usual signs of dehydration may be difficult to appreciate.

Hypernatraemia is a common feature of dehydration of acute onset and is commonly associated with a convulsive encephalopathy. This usually occurs during the process of rehydration and is probably due to water intoxication of the brain cells. However, the incidence of hypernatraemic dehydration seems to be declining in Britain, possibly due to several factors including (i) safer feeding practices with correctly mixed feeds, (ii) use of the newer modified milks during health, and (iii) avoidance of incorrect sugar or salt solutions during the illness.

Respiratory tract

Upper respiratory tract infections occur in about 20 per cent of cases and occasionally this may progress to a severe bronchopneumonia.

Venous thrombosis

Venous thrombosis of the cerebral cortical veins and more rarely of the renal veins, may complicate prolonged or severe gastroenteritis. Cortical vein thrombosis, which is often fatal, presents with convulsions, cranial nerve lesions, a bulging fontanelle and blood staining of the CSF.

Dietary intolerance

Not infrequently, after an initial partial recovery, there is a return of diarrhoea when milk feeds are re-introduced. This is most often due to malabsorption of lactose and sometimes also of sucrose. The stools become watery and may be quite acidic (pH below 5) containing an excess of reducing substances (0·5 per cent or more) which can be demonstrated by the clinitest method. Transient gluten-intolerance and cows' milk intolerance may also develop at the same time.

Occasionally, a toddler who is otherwise well may continue to pass 2 or 3 large loose stools a day containing undigested foods such as peas and carrots. This is usually due to intestinal hurry and settles well with a low residue, finely-minced diet.

Diagnosis

Acute gastroenteritis must be distinguished from the following:

1 Dysentery or salmonella enteritis—the clinical illness may be

identical and is only distinguished by isolation of the causative organism from the faeces.

2 Parenteral infections accompanied by diarrhoea and vomiting, particularly those of the respiratory tract, the ears, the meninges and the urinary tract.

3 Haemolytic-uraemic syndrome.

4 Surgical diseases, particularly intussusception, occasionally appendicitis or even congenital pyloric stenosis.

More protracted gastroenteritis must be distinguished from the following:

1 Feeding mismanagement.

2 *Giardia lamblia* enteritis—this is a mild chronic protozoal enteritis which is common in children's nurseries.

3 Malabsorption diseases, including coeliac disease and cystic fibrosis. Coeliac disease usually presents insidiously with loose, bulky motions between the ages of one and five years. With the present trend towards the earlier introduction of cereals into the diet of infants, cases are being seen increasingly at a much earlier age, often with an acute diarrhoeal onset which requires careful differentiation from acute gastroenteritis.

4 The more permanent forms of lactose or other carbohydrate intolerance (genetically determined) or cows' milk protein intolerance.

5 Congenital megacolon—presenting with overflow diarrhoea.

Prognosis
Most deaths are due to dehydration. Grade 3 dehydration is about 50 per cent fatal and Grade 2 about one per cent. Premature infants or those suffering from previous illness or defect have a worse prognosis. The mortality in cases admitted to hospital is 1–2 per cent but in the event of a severe hospital epidemic, the mortality reaches 10–20 per cent. In England the mortality from gastroenteritis in children under two years of age has fallen from an average of 400 deaths per year to a present 100 deaths per year over the last 10 years. Usually recovery is complete, but hypernatraemic encephalopathy may cause permanent brain damage.

Treatment
Domiciliary management
Mild cases may be treated simply by the reduction in amount

and strength of milk feeds for a day or two until the symptoms settle.

In more marked cases, milk feeds are withdrawn and are replaced with feeds of an electrolyte solution of about half strength. A home-made solution of half-strength normal saline (4·5 g/litre or approximately a half level teaspoon of common salt to a pint of water) flavoured with orange is suitable but is not immediately popular with mothers. A flavoured effervescent solution tablet containing sodium and potassium chloride and sodium bicarbonate is generally available (Electrosol tablets) and makes a suitable replacement fluid when one tablet is dissolved in 125 ml (4 fluid ounces) of water. These fluids may be used for 2–3 days without biochemical control but it is important that the solutions are accurately made up. The solutions are given in amounts of 150 ml per kg body weight per day, divided into many small feeds spread over the day at hourly or at the most two-hourly intervals. If individual feeds are kept below 100 ml (3 fluid ounces), vomiting does not usually continue: in fact if vomiting does persist on this type of regime the diagnosis of gastroenteritis should be reconsidered. Dilute milk feeds may be restarted in 2–3 days, in smaller amounts and at shorter intervals initially, and a return to normal feeding is usually possible in a further 3–4 days in graduated steps.

Common mistakes which may aggravate the course of the disease are:

1   The withholding of all fluids in an attempt to improve the symptoms by 'starving' the baby.

2   The use of thickened feeds when normal milk feeds are being vomited.

3   (Most important of all), the use of glucose solutions as a replacement fluid. Glucose is highly soluble and the mother commonly prepares a hypertonic solution, which will draw water from the body into the gut and aggravate the diarrhoea and vomiting. Commercial effervescent liquid glucose preparations are similarly unsuitable.

Antibiotics appear to play little or no part in the management of gastroenteritis, unless an associated infection such as otitis media or other respiratory tract infection is present. There are a number of antidiarrhoeal drugs or preparations advertised, but these do not appear to influence the course of the disease.

Hospital management

Severe cases, where the diarrhoea is very frequent or watery or where signs of dehydration appear, are better treated in hospital, where they are strictly isolated. The most important aspect of treatment is the replacement of water and electrolyte losses and antibiotics and antidiarrhoeal drugs are not normally used. Repeated serum electrolyte, blood pH and bicarbonate estimations, together with daily weighing are important guides to the success of treatment.

Apart from the normal fluid requirement of 150 ml per kg per day, an additional fluid increment is necessary for the first 24–48 hours to replace the fluid losses of dehydration. This increment is based on the clinical grading of dehydration and the corresponding weight loss which varies from 2·5 to 10 per cent of body weight. This is the equivalent of a fluid loss of 25–100 ml per kg per day. Therefore the total amount of fluid replacement in dehydration varies from 175 to 250 ml per kg per day depending on the clinical grade.

The composition of the replacement fluid cannot be deduced from the serum electrolytes as the serum sodium varies from very high to very low and the serum potassium does not reflect the true body loss of potassium. Therefore replacement fluids tend to be based on the composition of the actual fluid loss, essentially that of diarrhoeal fluid. Suitable replacement fluids include half-strength Darrow's solution, half-strength normal saline and Electrosol tablet solution.

When severe acidosis is present, extra bicarbonate is added to the replacement fluid, using 8·4 per cent sodium bicarbonate solution which contains 1 meq bicarbonate per ml.

When the serum sodium is above 150 mEq/litre, fluids of greater than half-strength are normally used, as otherwise, too rapid lowering of the serum sodium may precipitate a rapid shift of water into the cells to lower the intracellular osmolarity correspondingly. This may cause a convulsive encephalopathy. In hypernatraemia, fluid is given more slowly than the calculated rate, and frequently by mouth, for the same reasons.

Most cases of Grades 1 and 2 dehydration may be rapidly and safely rehydrated with oral fluids. Repeated feeds of 30–60 ml may be given without provoking vomiting. Initially feeds may be given every 15–30 minutes for 2–3 hours, after which hourly feeds are given until the day's fluid requirements are complete. In most cases, improvement begins within an hour or two and dehydration is completely relieved within 24 hours. If vomiting persists or improvement is not seen within 1–2 hours, the same type and amounts of fluid (brought up to normal strength with glucose) is given intravenously. These regimes require special nursing and close medical supervision during the early critical hours of treatment.

Grade 3 dehydration requires urgent intravenous fluid therapy to relieve the peripheral circulatory failure. Plasma may be used as the initial fluid, changing to half-strength Darrow's solution when the shock is relieved.

When the dehydration is completely relieved and the symptoms are settling, quarter-strength milk feeds are reintroduced with a gradual return to normal feeding in the ensuing few days.

When lactose intolerance is suspected, the ordinary milk feeds are replaced by a low-lactose milk such as Galactomin. Because of the not infrequent concurrence of transient cows' milk protein and gluten intolerance it may be better to commence feeding with a formula such as Pregestimil which contains glucose, medium chain triglycerides and altered casein. These dietary restrictions need only continue for a few weeks in most cases.

Sometimes, the child is intolerant to all forms of oral feeding. This is seen particularly in the severe hospital epidemic type of gastroenteritis. In such cases, a period of total intravenous alimentation with glucose, amino acid and fat preparations is necessary.

Prevention

Breast feeding is an important preventive measure in the first three months of life. Improvements in the social, medical, nutritional and hygienic standards of a country are invariably accompanied by a decreased incidence and mortality from gastroenteritis.

In the event of a severe hospital epidemic, the spread of infection may be limited by an agreed policy to treat all recognized cases in a single designated unit which should be completely separate from any hospital containing other baby units. Admissions to infected wards are stopped and transfers between wards or hospitals are kept to an absolute minimum.

F*

CHAPTER 28

Miscellaneous Gastrointestinal Infections

1 Cholera

Cholera is an acute gastrointestinal infection due to *Vibrio cholerae*. The disease is endemic in parts of Asia, particularly the Ganges basin, but from time to time epidemics have spread throughout the world. The classical non-haemolytic *V. cholerae* (Inaba and Ogawa serotypes) was probably responsible for the great world pandemics of the nineteenth century. These organisms are excreted in very large numbers during the acute illness, but the carrier state is rare. After excretion the organism may survive in water or wet textiles for one to two weeks.

In recent years the related haemolytic El Tor vibrio (also Inaba and Ogawa serotypes), originally endemic in Indonesia, became more widely prevalent and reached Europe in 1971 but this epidemic is now subsiding. The El Tor vibrio may continue to be excreted for up to three months after the acute illness and this increases the likelihood of spread of infection. In the last year epidemic cholera has been common in the Middle East. Since 1970 there have been 20 confirmed cases in Britain, mostly due to V. El Tor (Ogawa strain); all were imported.

Outbreaks of cholera are caused classically by the contamination of drinking water by human excreta. Food-borne transmission may also occur. Rapid spread of the infection from place to place is due to the movement of mild cases or symptomless excretors.

Clinical picture

The severe case presents acutely with the rapid onset of vomiting and continuous diarrhoea, accompanied by abdominal colic and leg cramps. The fluid loss may lead to peripheral circulatory failure (shock) and death within 24 hours. Cases with shock frequently develop acute renal failure. Milder cases and symptomless excretors have been increasingly recognized in recent years.

The essential treatment is the rapid intravenous replacement of the fluid losses. The organism is sensitive to a number of antibiotics, including tetracycline and this drug is often recommended. However, as with other intestinal tract infections, there is little clear evidence of the value of antibiotics.

The prevention of cholera depends mainly on the provision of pure water supplies and the safe sanitary disposal of excreta. It would be very difficult for cholera to spread following importation into a developed country. Cholera vaccine provides only partial protection for up to 6 months. The World Health Organization has withdrawn official recognition of the International Certificate of cholera vaccination because of its very doubtful value as a public health measure. However, as may countries, particularly in Africa and Asia still demand evidence of vaccination in travellers, the Certificate is still in widespread unofficial use. Cholera is one of the diseases kept under close surveillance by the World Health Organization.

2 Non-cholera vibrios
Recently in patients returning from tropical countries, acute diarrhoeal disease has been associated with non-cholera vibrios. These organisms are biochemically similar to *Vibrio cholerae* but are not agglutinated by cholera antiserum.

3 Campylobacter enteritis
Recent studies have shown that organisms of *Campylobacter* species are a common cause of acute enteritis in Britain. There are a large number of subtypes which are widely distributed among poultry, dogs and farm animals which may all be sources of infection. All age groups may be involved but the disease is most common in adults. Outbreaks have occurred following a common meal and spread has been noted within families, particularly between children and from children to their parents. Several milk-borne outbreaks have now been reported.

The illness often presents with fever lasting for several hours or days before the onset of diarrhoea which persists for several days but occasionally for 2–3 weeks. A minority of the patients have quite severe and prolonged abdominal pain or bloody diarrhoea.

The disease is diagnosed by the culture of the organism from the faeces and it is known that high antibody titres develop in the serum in convalescence. The organism is usually sensitive to erythromycin, tetracycline and chloramphenicol but not to ampicillin. However, the disease is self-limiting and, as with other bacterial intestinal infections, the value of antibiotics is doubtful.

4 Vibrio parahaemolyticus infection

These vibrios are widely distributed in Pacific Ocean sea-water and commonly cause gastroenteritis in countries like Japan following the ingestion of seafood. They have been responsible for several small food poisoning outbreaks in Britain, usually due to consumption of seafood, particularly crab, of Far Eastern origin. Recently the same organism has been found in British coastal waters.

5 Bacillus cereus enteritis

B. cereus is a spore-bearing, aerobic organism which has caused an increasing number of food poisoning outbreaks in recent years in Britain. Fried or boiled rice from Chinese restaurants has been implicated in most cases. It is common practice in such restaurants to boil large quantities of rice which is then stored at room temperature. This readily encourages the multiplication of *B. cereus* which may survive the final reheating stage and so give rise to acute food poisoning. There have also been recent reports of infection from milk, dried milk and pork pie. Two types of illness have been described, one of 1–5 hours incubation in which the emphasis is on vomiting and the other of 8–16 hours incubation in which diarrhoea and abdominal pain predominates.

6 Giardiasis

This is an infection of the small bowel caused by a flagellated protozoan, *Giardia lamblia*, which has a worldwide distribution. Infection is through the faecal-oral transmission of cysts passed by an infected case. Trophozoites develop from these cysts and colonize the upper small intestine sometimes causing mucosal damage. The infection remains asymptomatic in many cases but in others may cause chronic, protracted diarrhoea with fat malabsorption.

Giardiasis is an important cause of 'travellers' diarrhoea' and has been commonly reported in travellers to and from many temperate and tropical parts of the world. After an incubation period of about two weeks there is the acute onset of watery diarrhoea which settles in 1–2 weeks but may persist less severely for several months. The condition also occurs in this country particularly in young children and is common in residential nurseries. In these cases, the onset is less explosive and the usual picture is of a persistent mild diarrhoea with faulty fat absorption and failure to thrive. The condition may spread within a family or an institution.

The diagnosis is made by the microscopic identification of cysts or flagellated trophozoites in fresh faeces or of trophozoites in duodenal aspirate. Metronidazole (adult dose 2 g daily) is the treatment of choice.

7 Pseudomembranous colitis

This is a serious condition which may occur in middle-aged or elderly people who have undergone abdominal surgery and who have been treated with oral antibiotics. Although staphylococcal enterocolitis may occur in exactly similar circumstances it is now recognized that pseudomembranous colitis is due to overgrowth of certain uncommon strains of clostridia, particularly *Cl. difficile*, which excrete an exotoxin which causes inflammation and necrosis of the colonic mucosa with pseudomembrane formation. Many antibiotics can initiate the condition, but clindamycin is most commonly incriminated.

The condition presents with severe watery diarrhoea about 5–10 days after the antibiotic begins. The patient may deteriorate rapidly into dehydration and peripheral circulatory failure and the disease is commonly fatal.

The diagnosis may be suspected by the clinical circumstances, the absence of staphylococci in the faeces and the sigmoidoscopic appearances. Confirmation depends on the detection of clostridial toxin in the faeces in HeLa cell tissue cultures.

The patient requires energetic treatment with intravenous fluids to correct dehydration and restore the circulation. Nutrition must be maintained with intravenous aminoacid preparations such as Aminoplex 5. The initial antibiotic is withdrawn and there are reports the corticosteroids used as in acute ulcerative colitis and vancomycin are beneficial.

CHAPTER 29

Dehydration

Dehydration is the clinical and biochemical state which results from excess loss of water and electrolytes from the body. In gastrointestinal infections, the fluid loss is from vomiting and diarrhoea, the latter usually causing the greater loss. There is considerable variation in the composition of diarrhoeal fluid but the following figures may be taken as the average electrolyte content, with the normal serum or extracellular fluid (ECF) level shown for comparison.

	Sodium (mmol/l)	Potassium (mmol/l)	Chloride (mmol/l)	Bicarbonate (mmol/l)
Diarrhoeal fluid	70	30	50	approx. 20
Serum (ECF)	150	5	100	25

(a) Sodium and chloride changes

Diarrhoeal fluid contains about half the serum content of sodium and chloride. Therefore the abrupt loss of large amounts of hypotonic sodium chloride solution from the body frequently leads to a rise in the serum sodium and chloride levels through a relatively greater loss of water; this is referred to as hypernatraemia. So despite the loss of large amounts of sodium from the body, the serum sodium may reach very high levels (152–180 mmol/l). Infants with acute diarrhoea are particularly liable to develop hypernatraemic dehydration because (a) they have a relatively larger body surface area leading to greater insensible water loss; this is more evident in obese and febrile infants, (b) the immature kidney is unable to conserve water as efficiently as in adults, particularly if the function is already stretched to the limit by the use of concentrated feeds which increase the renal solute load. Infants with more protracted diarrhoea tend to develop hyponatraemia, whereas in adult patients dehydration is either normonatraemic or hyponatraemic.

In hypernatraemic states, there is concurrent hypertonicity of the intracellular fluid because of the shift of water from the cells into the hypertonic ECF. If the hypernatraemic case is treated rapidly with dilute fluids, there will be a precipitate fall in the serum (ECF) sodium. This will result in a large shift of water into the intracellular fluid to reduce the tonicity and thereby retain the balance between the fluid compartments. This may have the serious clinical consequence of encephalopathy due to water intoxication of the brain cells.

(b) Potassium changes

The potassium content of diarrhoeal fluid is several times higher than the serum (ECF) level. The main body reservoir of potassium is the intracellular fluid, so that the high level in diarrhoea fluid is presumably due to cellular disruption in the bowel and to an excess secretion of mucus which has a high potassium content. The loss of these large amounts of potassium is not at first reflected in the serum (ECF) level which remains normal. Later the serum potassium will fall, but this will signify a much greater loss of potassium from the cells. In protracted diarrhoea, there is often a cumulative loss of potassium and the serum potassium will eventually fall to very low levels. This is a dangerous condition leading to muscular hypotonia and cardiac dysrhythmias. Theoretical calculations of the potassium deficit, based on the serum (ECF) levels always give a serious under-estimate of the actual body loss. Replacement fluids often contain 20–40 mmol/l potassium, and this is safe if renal function is normal.

(c) Acid–base changes

Diarrhoeal fluid has a high bicarbonate content and as the loss from this source is usually much greater than the loss of acid gastric contents, the pH of the blood falls and a metabolic acidosis develops. Severe acidosis is in itself dangerous, producing pallor, hypotension and rapid, gasping respirations. The bicarbonate deficit may be estimated from the following formula:

Bicarbonate deficit = $(24 - \text{standard HCO}_3)$
(mmol/l) $\times \text{ECF (litres)} \times 2$

The theoretical calculation always gives a considerable under-estimate and as shown in the formula may be multiplied by 2. If the replacement fluid in use does not contain sufficient bicarbonate (or lactate) to replace the deficit, further sodium bicarbonate 8·4 per cent solution (1 mmol per ml) may be added. The ECF volume (litres) is roughly equal to one third of the body weight (kg).

(d) Renal function

The blood urea rises in most cases of dehydration. In infancy this is usually due to pre-renal causes due to the water loss and acute renal failure is very rare even when there has been a period of peripheral circulatory failure. In adults a period of hypotension frequently precipitates acute renal failure. A useful indication of the presence of established renal failure is the urinary urea/blood urea ratio which usually drops below 10 in renal failure, whereas in pre-renal uraemia the ratio remains above 20.

If renal failure is present, rehydration is carried out cautiously and fluid is stopped when the circulation is fully restored and hydration improved. Then a conservative water-restricted high-calorie low-protein regime is instituted. If diuresis does not occur with this regime and the blood urea reaches 45 mmol/l or the potassium 6·5 mmol/l then peritoneal dialysis is necessary and may be repeated until diuresis occurs. At this stage a high fluid and electrolyte intake is necessary to avoid a further episode of dehydration.

CHAPTER 30

Bacterial Meningitis

Many different bacteria are capable of causing meningitis, as is shown by the following list, which is arranged in the order of frequency of occurrence.

1 *Neisseria meningitidis*
2 *Haemophilus influenzae*
3 *Streptococcus pneumoniae*

4   *Mycobacterium tuberculosis*
5   Less common causes such as *E. coli*; haemolytic streptococci; *Listeria monocytogenes*; *Staph. aureus* and proteus species.

Meningococcal infection

This is a severe acute infectious disease, characterized by an
initial septicaemia, usually followed by pyogenic meningitis. A
purpuric skin rash is common.

Epidemiology

The disease is endemic throughout the world, with epidemics
occurring at irregular intervals. Large epidemics are almost an
annual event in some tropical countries particularly in Africa.
The two largest epidemics in Britain occurred during each
World War, probably due to the unusual overcrowded con-
centrations of young people. In the 1940 epidemic there were
12 700 cases, with a 20 per cent mortality.

The causative organism is *Neisseria meningitidis*, which is
classified in Groups A, B, C, X, Y, Z and W135. All groups may
cause similar disease, although the majority of cases in Britain
are now due to Group B. The source of infection is the
nasopharynx of a carrier, and the carrier rate in contacts may
be 25 per cent or higher when a case occurs. However, recent
surveys of carriers have shown a substantial proportion of
untypable organisms, which are probably nonpathogenic. The
great majority of carriers are asymptomatic, and the carrier
state is transient although immunity develops. Direct case-to-
case spread is unusual except in large families or institutions.
The disease spreads by droplet infection. The disease is most
common in poor and overcrowded communities and in residential institutions. There is a seasonal increase in winter and
spring, and possibly the prevalence of catarrhal upper respiratory infections facilitates the carrier state.

Although it can occur at any age, the disease is commonest in
children under five years old.

Pathology

The disease starts as a septicaemia, and, in fact, both acute
fulminating and chronic benign forms of septicaemia can occur

without meningitis. Commonly, however, invasion of the meninges follows the septicaemia. Occasionally other tissues, such as the joints and ears, are invaded during the septicaemic stage.

Incubation period
This is 1–3 days, with a limit of 1 week.

Clinical picture
The disease starts abruptly with pyrexia, malaise and prostration, accompanied by severe headache and vomiting. Young children are commonly irritable and restless. In 24–48 hours, the patient becomes drowsy and mentally confused, soon progressing to coma, occasionally accompanied by convulsions. A rash is present in half the cases. This usually consists of irregular petechiae of varying size scattered over the whole body; occasionally the rash consists of small erythematous papules with a petechial centre.

The main clinical sign of meningitis is rigidity of the muscles of the neck and spine, similar in mechanism to the rigidity of the abdominal muscles in peritonitis. The rigidity of the neck is present even in an unconscious patient, and is not strictly related to headache, although this symptom is usually present.

The recognition of minor degrees of neck rigidity requires considerable experience, since a headache due to febrile illness is aggravated by full flexion of the neck. Normally the spine can be flexed so that the head can touch the bent-up knees, but restriction of this movement occurs with meningeal irritation. The indirect signs described by Kernig and Brudzinski are of limited value in detecting or assessing meningeal irritation.

In infants, the presence of neck and spinal rigidity is difficult to elicit, but tense bulging of the anterior fontanelle is an important sign of meningeal irritation; this sign is found even when vomiting has caused some dehydration in the infant. Difficulty occurs in the examination of babies who are crying because the neck is then held rigid and the fontanelle bulges.

Fulminating septicaemia (Waterhouse–Friderichsen syndrome)
This is a rare and rapidly fatal presentation. The patient quickly becomes very ill, with pallor, hypotension and peripheral circulatory failure. Simultaenously, large and rapidly-spreading areas

of purpura appear in the skin, over the whole body. The temperature is normal or subnormal in most cases. There are usually no signs of meningitis and the CSF is normal, although blood culture is positive for *N. meningitidis*. Children under the age of two are most commonly affected. The whole course of the disease is rapid, and death can occur within a few hours of the onset.

Although adrenal haemorrhage is sometimes found at autopsy, the clinical picture is probably caused by septicaemic shock and disseminated intravascular coagulation (DIC) rather than by adrenal failure.

Chronic septicaemia
This condition, described in the 1940 epidemic, presented with bouts of pyrexia occurring every few days, recurrent rashes, resembling erythema nodosum, and recurrent joint pain and swelling. Blood culture was positive, and the illness persisted for many weeks. This condition is now very rare.

Complications
The following complications occur, but are uncommon:

Deafness
About five per cent of cases have some permanent impairment of hearing in one or both ears, due to a labyrinthitis.

Cranial nerve paralysis
This is usually a transient complication, and may affect the 3rd, 4th, 6th or 7th cranial nerves.

Hydrocephalus
This is due to organization of purulent exudate in the CSF pathway, commonly at the base of the brain. In the untreated disease, this was commonplace among survivors, but with modern treatment it has become rare.

Polyarthritis
This is a rare occurrence, and does not leave permanent joint damage, in spite of the presence of considerable effusion.

Pericarditis
This also occurs rarely.

Diagnosis

Meningococcal infection must be distinguished from:

1   Purpuric conditions including Weil's Disease, Henoch Schonlein purpura, thrombocytopenic purpura, leukaemia and blood dyscrasias, rare fulminating purpuric forms of viral infections such as measles and smallpox.

2   Febrile conditions such as otitis media, tonsillitis, upper lobe pneumonia and pyelitis, which may be accompanied by meningism (signs of meningeal irritation, without actual meningitis).

3   Other bacterial and viral forms of meningitis, by examination of the CSF.

4   Subarachnoid haemorrhage, by examination of the CSF which shows uniform bloodstaining, with a xanthochromic supernatant fluid.

N. meningitidis can be isolated from the blood in many cases. Examination of the CSF will show a polymorph count of 500–5000 cells, a raised protein of about 2–5 g/litre and in most cases a low or absent sugar content. In the majority of cases the organism is seen in films as Gram-negative diplococci, often intracellular, and can be isolated on culture. *N. meningitidis* is the most delicate of the organisms causing bacterial meningitis so that the finding of a sterile CSF is not uncommon. In this circumstance, the diagnosis may be confirmed by the demonstration of bacterial antigen in the CSF by cross-over immunoelectrophoresis. Further confirmation of the diagnosis may be obtained from rising serum antibody titres by the indirect haemagglutination method. These antigen and antibody tests are usually available in regional reference laboratories.

Prognosis

The untreated disease had a mortality of 65 per cent with a high morbidity among the survivors. Sulphonamides reduced the mortality in the 1940 epidemic to 20 per cent. The overall mortality is now 5–10 per cent. In young healthy adults the mortality may be as low as one per cent.

The fulminating septicaemic type is very often fatal. In established meningitis, the prognosis depends greatly on the level of consciousness of the patient. In conscious patients, death is rare; most fatalities occur in patients who are already unconscious at the time of diagnosis.

Treatment

Since the emergence of sulphonamide-resistant meningococci, penicillin is now regarded as the drug of choice. Approximately 10 per cent of the strains isolated in Britain are now resistant to sulphonamides and in Scotland the percentage is much higher. Penicillin should be given parenterally and in high doses. It penetrates the blood–brain barrier poorly in normal dosage, but when given in doses of 2 mega units every 4 hours, a reliable bactericidal level is rapidly found in the CSF and intrathecal administration is unnecessary. This high dose of penicillin may be reduced when the temperature returns to normal and the patient's condition improves, usually in 2–3 days. Treatment is continued for a week. In areas of low sulphonamide resistance, oral sulphadiazine may usefully be given in addition as this may allow discontinuation of penicillin injections when the sensitivity results become available.

In the fulminating septicaemic case, intravenous plasma, large doses of intravenous hydrocortisone (600–1200 mg daily) and oxygen are given, in addition to massive doses of penicillin, but in spite of this the condition is very often fatal. Because of the underlying intravascular coagulation heparin has been suggested as additional treatment, but no practical assessment of this has been made. Treatment should not be delayed while attempts to confirm the diagnosis are made, in fact the general practitioner should give large doses of penicillin and corticosteroids before the patient is transferred to hospital.

Prevention

At present meningococcal infection is an uncommon endemic disease, and little can be done to prevent the sporadic occurrence. Family and school contacts are commonly carriers. A two-day course of sulphonamide will usually clear the carrier state if the organism is sensitive, otherwise rifampicin or minocycline may be used. The routine treatment of contacts is more valuable in large families and in institutions. Quarantine of contacts is unnecessary. In epidemic times in institutions, adequate bed spacing and ventilation are important, and the prophylactic use of sulphonamides is worthwhile. Trials with group A and C vaccines, using capsular polysaccharide have given good results. Unfortunately it has not yet proved possible to produce a potent group B vaccine, the predominant organism in Britain.

Haemophilus meningitis

Epidemiology

This disease is endemic throughout the world. Cases may occur at any age, but are most common in the first five years of life. Case to case spread does not occur. The causative organism is a capsulated *H. influenzae* of Pittman type b., which is found occasionally in the nasopharynx of healthy people. Possibly as the consequence of an upper respiratory infection the organism enters the bloodstream, and hours or days later invades the meninges, causing a pyogenic meningitis. Other organs are not usually involved except occasionally the bones.

Clinical picture

The disease often presents rather insidiously, with a period of pyrexia and malaise lasting several days, before headache, vomiting and prostration appear. The signs of meningeal irritation are then usually, but not invariably, present. The patient will become drowsy, and eventually comatose, sometimes with convulsions and cranial nerve paralysis.

The diagnosis is confirmed by lumbar puncture, which shows a purulent CSF, with a high protein and low sugar content. The Gram film will usually show Gram-negative bacilli, which may be swarming or scanty, and the culture grows *H. influenzae*. The blood culture is frequently positive.

Complications such as cranial nerve palsies and hydrocephalus may occur, particularly where treatment has been delayed. Subdural effusion may occur and should be suspected when a child remains febrile and irritable with a tense bulging fontanelle but with an improving CSF picture. Diagnosis is confirmed by subdural tap, which is performed daily until no further fluid is obtained.

Treatment

Chloramphenicol remains the drug of choice. Satisfactory blood levels are obtained after oral administration and the drug penetrates the blood–brain barrier readily. So far, chloramphenicol-resistant strains have been reported only very rarely. It is given by intramuscular or intravenous injection for the first 48 hours, since vomiting may interfere with administration, and also because the absorption of the oral liquid palmitate from the gut is not reliable in children. The adult dose is 2 g daily, whilst the dose for a child is 50–100 mg/kg body weight, daily. Treatment is continued for 9–10 days as shorter courses have occasionally been followed by a relapse. Ampicillin is also effective and its lack of toxicity is an advantage. However, the drug has to be given in very large doses (400 mg/kg daily) by intravenous infusion and in recent years the emergence of ampicillin resistant *H. influenza* has detracted from the value of this drug. Effective treatment has reduced the mortality from 90 per cent to less than 10 per cent. In a minority of treated cases there is persistent neurological damage but the majority recover completely. No measures are effective in preventing the disease.

Pneumococcal meningitis

Epidemiology
Although less common than the two previous types of meningitis, pneumococcal meningitis is a more severe disease with a persistently high mortality. The *Strep. pneumoniae* may reach the meninges from the bloodstream, either from an existing respiratory tract infection or from an unknown source. In some cases, the infection reaches the meninges from a chronic otitis media, or via a congenital defect or fracture of the skull. The disease is not infectious. Although it is most common in children, it occurs at all ages and is the commonest type of bacterial meningitis in the over-50 age group.

Clinical picture
The illness starts acutely with pyrexia, headache and vomiting, progressing in 1 or 2 days to drowsiness and coma, with variable cranial nerve lesions and convulsions. The usual signs of meningeal irritation are found, the patient looks pale and ill, and has a low blood pressure. Blood culture may also be positive.

Lumbar puncture shows a purulent CSF, with high protein and low or absent sugar. The organism is usually abundant on a film, appearing as Gram-positive diplococci, and can be isolated on culture.

Otitis media is looked for, and any history of recent head injury noted. During convalescence, skull X-rays are necessary to exclude congenital defect or fracture.

Treatment

Because of the persistent mortality of from 20–40 per cent in this disease, the most energetic treatment is necessary to eliminate the organism as rapidly as possible. Intramuscular penicillin is given in a dosage of 4 mega units every 2 hours, until definite clinical improvement begins, when the dosage is reduced to 2 mega units every 4 hours until the temperature is normal and the CSF sterile on two successive days. In addition, full doses of sulphadimidine are given by mouth. There is diminishing enthusiasm for the use of intrathecal penicillin, because of erratic absorption and possible convulsive effects, but this form of therapy may be given once, at the onset, in a dose of 10,000 units. Treatment is continued for 10 days. Cephaloridine in a daily dose of 100 mg/kg up to 6 g daily in eight-hourly intramuscular injections along with alternate day intrathecal dose of 50 mg is a suitable alternative.

Some cases in coma sustain irreversible brain damage and die days or weeks after the onset of the illness, in spite of the eradication of the infection and a return of the CSF to normal.

Where an otitis or skull fracture is found, after recovery, the patient is referred to the appropriate specialist surgeon, as operative treatment may be possible, and may prevent recurrence of the disease.

Less common forms of pyogenic meningitis*

E. coli meningitis occurs as a primary disease only during the neonatal period. It is a severe disease with a high mortality. In this age group the usual signs of meningitis are often lacking, and the only signs may be pallor, irritability, vomiting and failure to feed and thrive.

Most other forms of meningitis (streptococcal, staphylococcal, proteus group, etc.) are secondary to head injury; congenital defects such as meningocoele; otitis media or septicaemic infection. The illness is severe, and the infection tends to localize, giving rise to subdural effusions, septic phlebitis of the cranial venous sinuses, or the formation of a brain abscess.

Group B haemolytic streptococci have recently emerged as an important cause of severe and often fatal neonatal septicaemia and meningitis, the infection originating from the genital tract of the mother.

*For *Tuberculous meningitis* see Chapter 31.

CHAPTER 31

Tuberculosis

This is a chronic infectious disease caused by *Mycobacterium tuberculosis*. The commonest and most infectious form of the disease is chronic pulmonary tuberculosis, but many more acute varieties are encountered.

Epidemiology and pathology

M. tuberculosis exists as two main strains, the human and the bovine. The main source of infection of the human strain is the respiratory tract of an 'open' case of adult pulmonary tuberculosis. Transmission takes place by droplet infection or by close personal contact. The initial exposure of a child to such infection results in primary tuberculosis. The first manifestation of this condition is the formation of a small sub-pleural lesion termed the Ghon focus, and from this lesion, infection spreads rapidly to the lymph glands at the hilum of the lung, this combination is known as the primary complex. These glands enlarge with granulomatous inflammatory changes which may undergo caseation. In the majority of cases the infection heals spontaneously in a few weeks or months, the glands regress and may calcify. During the primary infection, the body tissues become sensitized to tuberculo-protein, so that an intradermal injection of tuberculin produces a red indurated reaction, which reaches its maximum in three days. This is the basis of the tuberculin or Mantoux test which becomes positive about six weeks after the onset of the primary infection, and is associated with the development of immunity to infection. About eight per cent of schoolchildren now have a positive tuberculin reaction (by Heaf test) at the age of 13 years, but even in this small percentage it is considered that the milder positive reactions (Heaf test Grade 1) are non-specific and should be recorded as negative. In a minority of cases of primary tuberculosis, infection spreads from the hilar lymph glands:
1   To a bronchus, causing a segmental lung lesion.
2   By lymphatics, causing pleurisy with effusion.

3   By the bloodstream causing:
(a) Miliary tuberculosis.
(b) Tuberculous meningitis.
(c) Metastic infection in kidney, adrenal, bone, joint, etc., producing localized chronic disease.

The main source of bovine tuberculosis is the milk of infected cows. In this type of infection, the primary lesion is situated in the tonsil, or Peyer's patches with spread to the cervical or mesenteric lymph glands. Occasionally, infection spreads to bone, joint or peritoneum. Bovine tuberculosis is now largely eradicated.

In a tuberculin-positive adult, a small dose of the infecting organism is dealt with by immune processes, but a large infecting dose may cause a local inflammatory reaction in the lung, which may lead to progressive disease with cavity formation and infectious sputum. Close and prolonged contact with infection in a family or classroom frequently leads to multiple cases of the disease. Certain groups of people possess a poor natural resistance to tuberculosis: amongst these are the Irish, Scots, Indians and Pakistanis; on the other hand, Jews possess a higher natural resistance.

Clinical picture

1   Primary tuberculosis of the lung
This infection is often entirely asymptomatic, but the child may be unwell for a few weeks, with a poor appetite, dry cough and evening pyrexia. There are usually no abnormal physical signs in the chest. The diagnosis is established by the discovery of unilateral hilar gland enlargement on chest X-ray. The tuberculin test is positive, and sometimes *M. tuberculosis* can be cultured from morning gastric lavage specimens.

Occasionally, erosion of a bronchus produces a distal segmental lesion which may vary from segmental aspiration collapse, which quickly resolves, to caseating pneumonitis, which heals by fibrosis, leaving an area of bronchiectasis. Chest X-ray shows a wedge opacity related to the hilum, in any lobe, most commonly the right middle lobe.

2   Miliary tuberculosis
This may occur during the primary infection, or months or years afterwards. The patient presents with fever, tiredness and

sweating, commonly with a dry cough and shortness of breath.
Over a period of 2 or 3 weeks, the patient's condition de-
teriorates steadily; there is increasing fever, dyspnoea and rapid
loss of weight. Physical examination often reveals fine crepitations at the bases of the lungs, and a palpable spleen. The
appearance of choroidal tubercles is diagnostic of miliary
tuberculosis and suggests an accompanying meningitis; these are
circular yellow areas, fading at the edge into normal retina, and
a quarter of the size of the optic disc. The tuberculin test is
usually positive, and chest X-ray shows diffuse fine nodulation,
the 'snowstorm lung'. *M. tuberculosis* can usually be isolated
from sputum, bronchial lavage or gastric lavage.

3 Tuberculous meningitis

This may be an early or late complication of primary tuberculosis, or may accompany miliary or chronic pulmonary tuberculosis. The onset is insidious with mild recurrent headache,
slight malaise, irritability and moodiness, and occasional mild
pyrexia. After one or two weeks the patient's condition de-
teriorates, there is more severe headache and pyrexia, and more
obvious mental and personality changes, which may take the
form of drowsiness, lack of attention, mild confusion and
euphoria. At this time, neck and spinal rigidity gradually appear
and cranial nerve lesions particularly of the 6th and 3rd nerves
occur. During the 3rd or 4th week, drowsiness gradually
deepens to coma, and there are often major neurological
changes such as spastic hemiplegia or diplegia. The tuberculin
test is positive, and chest X-ray shows evidence of active
tuberculosis in a minority of cases. Examination of the CSF
reveals a pleocytosis of 100–750 cells, mostly lymphocytes. The
protein is raised to $1–5 \, g/l$ (100–500 mg per cent), and the sugar
is usually reduced to below $1 \cdot 6 \, mmol/l$ (30 mg per cent). Acid-
fast bacilli can be seen in Ziehl–Neelsen stained CSF deposit in
about a quarter of the cases, and can be isolated by culture or
preferably by guinea-pig inoculation in the majority of cases.
The radioactive bromide partition test may provide confirmation by showing a drop in the blood/CSF bromide ratio to
less than $1 \cdot 6$ in cases of tuberculous meningitis. (Normal ratio 2
or over.)

4 Tuberculous pleurisy

This usually occurs months or years after the primary infection.

Although the onset may be insidious, characteristically the illness is a stormy one with high fever, cough, dyspnoea and pleuritic pain; in the early stages it is often mistaken for pneumonia. The physical signs of a moderate or large pleural effusion are found: percussion dullness, absent vocal fremitus and diminished breath sounds, with a strip of bronchial breathing at the upper border of the fluid. The tuberculin test is always positive and chest X-ray confirms the presence of an effusion. On aspiration, the fluid is clear and straw coloured and contains mainly lymphocytes with very few pus cells or mesothelial cells. *M. tuberculosis* is cultured from the fluid in about half the cases, and pleural biopsy confirms the diagnosis histologically in almost every case.

5   Adult pulmonary tuberculosis

This is the most common form of the disease. The onset may be insidious or may be more abrupt, often described as 'influenza which never cleared up completely'. Cough is present throughout the illness, dry at first, later productive of mucoid sputum with occasionally haemoptysis. There is increasing tiredness, the appetite becomes poor and there is usually a considerable loss of weight. Late in the illness 'night sweats occur', the patient wakens feeling weak and ill with the body and clothing soaked with sweat. These symptoms may persist for weeks or months before the patient seeks help, sometimes prompted by an alarming symptom such as haemoptysis.

Physical examination of the chest is unreliable and often reveals nothing. Chest X-ray shows infiltrative or fibrotic changes usually in one or both upper lobes, often with multiple cavities, the hallmark of pulmonary tuberculosis. The sputum is usually positive on direct ZN staining and is practically always culture positive; the disease is highly infectious at this stage.

The incidence of pulmonary tuberculosis has steadily diminished over the last 25 years, particularly since the advent of effective chemotherapy. The disease is still relatively common in certain groups including the elderly male 'bronchitic', the hostel-dweller and vagrant, and the Irish and Scots of Celtic origin.

6   Tuberculosis in the Asian immigrant

This has been a problem in Britain for the last 20 years. Asian immigrants have a poor natural resistance to tuberculosis and tend to develop a more acute disseminated type of disease, usually in their first few years in Britain.

A common presentation in the Asian patient is persistent fever lasting for days or weeks, where all investigations prove negative. In this circumstance a course of antituberculous chemotherapy is fully justified as a therapeutic trial and is frequently followed by rapid and complete recovery.

More usually the patient presents with fever and with evidence of disease in one or more systems. Lymph gland involvement is common, including the hilar, abdominal, neck or even axillary glands. Respiratory disease is common, sometimes with simultaneous involvement of the hilar glands, lungs and pleura. Miliary tuberculosis, meningitis, renal disease, abdominal disease (peritoneal, hepatic, intestinal) and bone disease are all encountered.

Although the patient presents with acute disease and often with involvement of multiple systems, there is usually a correspondingly rapid improvement and resolution on treatment with chemotherapy.

Tuberculosis has appeared in two waves among immigrants, firstly among young adults entering the country in large numbers in 1960–1965 and more recently a second wave in adolescent children arriving to join their parents in Britain. Once the immigrants have settled in Britain for a number of years, the incidence of tuberculosis falls markedly.

Treatment

The basis of treatment is the use of antituberculous drugs (see Table 8). The drugs are given in combination to prevent resistance and for a sufficient period of time (usually 9 months; maximum 12 months) to ensure a cure and prevent a relapse.

TABLE 8 Antituberculous drugs

Drug	Route	Adult dose	Children's dose
Isoniazid	Oral	300 mg daily	8 mg/kg daily
Rifampicin	Oral	600 mg daily	15 mg/kg daily
Ethambutol	Oral	15 mg/kg daily for 2 months then omit	
Streptomycin	Intramusc.	1 g daily	10–20 mg/kg daily

The most common combination is isoniazid, rifampicin and ethambutol for 2 months, after which ethambutol is omitted and the other two drugs continued for 7 months. Streptomycin may be used in place of ethambutol.

1 Primary tuberculosis

Cases with chest X-ray changes are treated with standard chemotherapy. In the absence of X-ray changes, any tuberculin-positive child under the age of 5 years who is a contact, is treated for 6–9 months with isoniazid and rifampicin. An older child contact who has a recent tuberculin conversion is similarly treated, to prevent the development of disease. The use of isoniazid alone in these circumstances is not justifiable.

2 Miliary tuberculosis

Triple chemotherapy is used and is continued without reduction until there is satisfactory clearing of the chest X-ray. Cortico-steroids are helpful in reducing the toxicity in severely-ill cases.

3 Tuberculous meningitis

Three or four standard drugs are used (normally including isoniazid and rifampicin which penetrate well into the CSF). Intrathecal treatment is now seldom used, although in a severe or late case daily intrathecal streptomycin may be given for four weeks (adult dose 100 mg, children 25–50 mg). There is evidence that corticosteroids are useful in preventing exudate formation, and in reducing oedema of the brain.

In patients who are conscious when treatment is started, the recovery rate is more than 90 per cent, and there are few sequelae. In unconscious cases, the recovery rate is about 60 per cent, and neurological and mental sequelae are common in the survivors.

4 Tuberculous pleurisy

Treatment with the standard drugs is essential, otherwise 25 per cent of the cases will develop progressive pulmonary tuber-culosis. Corticosteroids greatly accelerate the reabsorption of the pleural fluid, rendering repeated aspiration unnecessary, and reducing the incidence of late pleural thickening.

5 Chronic pulmonary tuberculosis—standard chemotherapy.

6   *Tuberculosis in Asian immigrants*—standard chemotherapy.

Prevention

1   Infectious cases are treated in hospital, until the sputum is negative on culture.

2   All types of tuberculosis are notifiable, and as a result, a search is made for cases among contacts in the home, at school and at work. The chest is X-rayed in all adult contacts. Children receive a tuberculin test and only positive reactors have an X-ray. Tuberculin-negative children are given BCG vaccine, after removal from contact with the infectious case. In rare circumstances when the tuberculin-negative young child cannot be removed from contact with the infectious case (normally the mother), the child may be vaccinated with a special isoniazid-resistant BCG strain, and thereafter given isoniazid by mouth as a prophylactic measure. Contacts are observed for a further year, and are advised to report immediately any illness.

3   General population surveys by Mass Miniature X-ray have been discontinued, but the examination of special groups such as immigrants, prisoners, patients in psychiatric institutions and patients referred because of chest symptoms continues to be worthwhile. An initial X-ray is necessary in special groups such as nurses, medical students and school teachers but routine repeat X-rays are no longer advocated.

4   Routine tuberculin testing, usually by Heaf or Tine method, is occasionally a useful diagnostic procedure in specific groups of children.

5   BCG is a live-attenuated vaccine, which is about 80 per cent effective in preventing tuberculosis. The vaccine is given by intradermal injection, and results in a small ulcerated lesion which persists for several weeks and leaves a characteristic punched-out scar. Tuberculin conversion is the rule, after BCG vaccination. The vaccine is recommended for general use in all tuberculin negative and also Heaf test Grade 1 positive children at 10–13 years of age. It is also used in special groups such as tuberculin-negative contacts, nurses and medical students. In underdeveloped countries BCG is recommended for all babies, but with the present degree of control of tuberculosis in this country, this practice is not justified. Babies born into a family containing a known case of tuberculosis are vaccinated at birth. Babies born of Asian immigrant parents may also be routinely

vaccinated at birth, because of the high incidence of tuberculosis in this group and the difficulty in case tracing. As the incidence of tuberculosis continues to fall and as the disease is largely curable, the use of BCG on a community basis becomes increasingly uneconomical. Furthermore, as increasing numbers of young people are tuberculin negative, the diagnostic value of the tuberculin test would increase were it not for the conversions due to BCG. For these reasons it may not be long before a more selective use of BCG is preferred to the present routine use. BCG vaccine is contraindicated if skin sepsis or chronic skin disease such as eczema is present. Other immunizations in the same arm should be avoided for 3 months after BCG.

6 Extensive pasteurization of milk and the eradication of the disease in cattle have virtually eliminated bovine tuberculosis in this country.

CHAPTER 32

Brucellosis

Organisms of the *Brucella* genus commonly cause infection of cattle, goats and pigs in many parts of the world and can be the cause of much acute, subacute and chronic disease in man.

The three main species of *Brucella* organisms and their principal animal reservoirs are *Br. abortus* (cattle), *Br. melitensis* (goat) and *Br. suis* (pig). Less common species are *Br. canis*, which affects dogs and can produce infection in laboratory workers handling dogs and *Br. ovis* (sheep). *Brucella melitensis* generally produces a more severe infection in man than either *Br. abortus* or *Br. suis* and is prevalent in communities dependent on goats for milk, as in the Mediterranean area. The only variety endemic in Britain is *Br. abortus* infection in cattle.

Brucella abortus infection

Epidemiology

Br. abortus is the cause of contagious abortion in cattle. Until recently the disease used to be widespread in Britain with about 30 per cent of herds showing some evidence of infection but the current estimates put this figure at 14 per cent, indicating encouraging progress of the *Brucella* eradication programme. *Brucella* organisms can remain viable for long periods outside the animal host but are easily killed by the pasteurization of milk. About four per cent of milk and two per cent of cream is still not heat-treated; this occurs mainly in the rural areas. Infection is through direct contact with tissues, blood, urine, vaginal discharges and parturition products from infected animals and also by the consumption of infected milk or milk products such as cream or cheese. Veterinary surgeons and farmers who handle cattle at parturition are particularly liable to infection which gains entry by alimentary or respiratory routes. Infection may occur in abattoir workers and in laboratory technicians. Case to case spread in humans is almost unknown. Although the incidence of the disease in cattle is high, in humans it is low and is difficult to assess accurately since the disease is not notifiable. There are about 200 diagnosed cases each year in England and Wales; probably much larger numbers of mild or subclinical cases occur. Surveys have shown serological evidence of infection in 1–20 per cent of the population in rural areas, with a very much higher incidence in selected groups such as dairy-farming communities (30 per cent) and veterinary surgeons (60–90 per cent). Clinical disease is most common in young adult males. After entering the body, the organisms localize in the reticulo-endothelial cells of the liver, spleen, bone marrow and lymph glands. Two factors are probably responsible for the development of the clinical disease—endotoxin production and the cell-mediated immune response.

Incubation period
This is difficult to determine but is probably 2–4 weeks.

Clinical picture
The disease is most variable both in severity and in clinical manifestations.

Mild cases often remain ambulant, with slight irregular pyrexia, headache and malaise which may last for several weeks. Severe cases present with fever, which usually persists for 4–8 weeks, but occasionally lasts for months or even years. The

G

fever may be punctuated by remissions and relapses, but a truly undulant pattern is more commonly a feature of *Br. melitensis* infection. Drenching sweats frequently accompany the fever. Other features are pain in the limbs, back and abdomen, flitting arthralgia or sore throat and persistent cough with signs of bronchitis. Neurological features include headache, irritability, depression and insomnia. Erythematous rashes may occur and there may be considerable loss of weight. Physical examination may show enlargement of the spleen, liver and lymph glands.

Rarely, cases run a severely toxic course, with haemorrhagic features.

A chronic form of brucellosis occurs with occasional low grade pyrexia, prolonged fatigue, tremor, depression, insomnia and varying rheumatic symptoms. This condition may be difficult to distinguish from psychoneurosis.

Complications include spondylitis and arthritis, usually affecting a single joint, meningo-encephalitis, peripheral neuritis, endocarditis, hepatitis and orchitis. These are much more common in *Br. melitensis* infections. Abortion does not occur in human brucellosis; this is because unlike the animal uterus, the human uterus does not contain erythritol, a potent growth stimulator of *Brucella* organisms.

Diagnosis

Confirmation of the diagnosis depends on laboratory investigations.

1 In a minority of cases, the organism is cultured from the blood or urine. It grows very slowly on special media in an atmosphere of carbon dioxide.

2 The most widely-used test is the demonstration of a raised or rising antibody titre by agglutination method. Titres of 1/80 or over are usually regarded as positive but most acute cases will have titres over 1/320. In chronic brucellosis, the agglutination test, which demonstrates IgM antibody, may become normal but IgG antibody persists and can be demonstrated by complement-fixation and Coombs anti-human globulin tests. The recently introduced radio-immunoassay of specific brucella immunoglobulin will help in problematic cases.

3 A positive brucellin intradermal test does not necessarily indicate active disease and is therefore valueless as a diagnostic test.

4 Blood counts usually show a leucopenia with a relative lymphocytosis.

Prognosis

The disease is rarely fatal. Most cases persist from 4 to 12 weeks, but the disease may run a prolonged and relapsing course in spite of antibiotic treatment.

Treatment

Tetracycline, in short courses, in a dose of 2 g daily produces a clinical remission, but relapses are common, probably due to the persistence of intracellular organisms. It is claimed that fewer relapses occur when tetracycline combined with streptomycin (1 g daily intramuscularly) is given for three weeks, followed by tetracycline alone for a further three weeks. Cotrimoxazole is an effective alternative.

Corticosteroids in conjunction with antibiotics are said to have a beneficial effect in severe or chronic cases.

The chronic-fatigued case with tremor may be helped by beta-adrenergic blocking drugs such as propranolol in small doses.

Prevention

An important preventive measure is the heat treatment of all cows' milk and cream. However, this eliminates only milk-borne infections and the elimination of human brucellosis can be achieved only by eradicating the animal reservoir of infection. To achieve this aim, the Ministry of Agriculture started in 1966 a *Brucella* eradication campaign to establish disease-free herds. This is being achieved by identifying infected herds followed by the slaughter and replacement of the infected animals. The scheme is working well, and by the end of 1975 two thirds of the United Kingdom herds were in the eradication scheme.

Other measures directed at reducing the reservoir of infection are:

1 Control over the disposal of infected cattle and carcases.

2 Search for the animal source in human cases.

3 Regular examination of milk samples by the ring test for brucella antibody will indicate which areas and which herds are infected.

4 When milk supplies are known to be infected, the Medical Officer for Environmental Health has the authority to enforce the heat treatment of milk.

5 The vaccination of calves with the S19 vaccine strain of *Br. abortus* provides some protection. However, a policy of vaccination is not presently favoured, as this would interfere with the skin and blood tests for the ascertainment of *Brucella*-free herds.

CHAPTER 33

Anthrax

Anthrax is normally a severe infection of domestic animals. Occasionally man acquires infection from an animal source, usually developing a cutaneous lesion or, rarely, a respiratory or gastrointestinal infection.

Epidemiology

The causative organism is *Bacillus anthracis*. Anthrax affects cattle, sheep and horses, and in these animals the infection usually takes the form of a fatal septicaemia. In the blood and tissues of such animals, the organism is present in its vegetative form, but on drying in aerobic conditions, highly resistant spores are formed, which remain viable for months or years. In Britain, animal anthrax is uncommon, but in India and Africa, where the disease is common, animal products are more likely to become infected. Thus, imported goods such as hides, wool and powdered bone meal, can carry the infection as spores. Although raw wool can be sterilized, animal hides cannot be disinfected without excessive damage. Most human cases in Britain result from contact with animal products, or with domestic animals, and so the disease is an occupational hazard among tannery workers, raw wool workers, veterinary surgeons, butchers, farmers and animal handlers. Cases have occurred in gardeners using infected bone meal as fertilizer and this is becoming an increasingly common source of infection. In man, cutaneous anthrax results from direct infection of a cut or abrasion or of apparently intact skin. The cutaneous lesion is infective until healed, but case-to-case spread is almost unknown. In Britain no case of respiratory or intestinal anthrax has been reported for several decades.

The pathological picture is an acute inflammatory reaction, with haemorrhagic necrosis, but without pus formation. From the cutaneous lesion, there is spread of infection to the regional lymph nodes, in some cases proceeding to a septicaemia.

Incubation period
Normally 1–3 days with limits of up to 7 days.

Clinical picture

Cutaneous anthrax
The old term 'malignant pustule' is a double misnomer since the lesion is not malignant and does not suppurate. Cutaneous anthrax usually occurs on the exposed skin such as the face, neck, hand or arm. The lesion starts as a small itching papule which develops in a few days to a thick-walled off-white vesicle with a dark red almost black base. Satellite lesions may develop round the original vesicle. There is surrounding erythema and striking local oedema. Over the course of a few days the vesicle ruptures leaving a dark red oozing granular base which slowly dries to a thick black crust which may persist for several weeks. The cutaneous lesion is usually painless. The lymph glands draining the area usually become enlarged and tender and on the limbs the red lines of an ascending lymphangitis are commonly seen. In some cases the lesion is not so well localized and a spreading cellulitis with gross oedema and superficial dark vesiculation occurs. In most cases there is fever and general malaise.

Septicaemia
In 10–20 per cent of cases of cutaneous anthrax, septicaemia develops and this more often follows lesions on the neck or face, or poorly localized extensive lesions. The patient will become seriously ill with high fever, prostration and falling blood pressure often with evidence of haemolytic jaundice and renal failure. Unless treated early, these cases are usually fatal.

Systemic anthrax—pulmonary or intestinal
Both forms are fortunately very rare, are not usually diagnosed

and are normally fatal. Pulmonary anthrax was formerly known as 'Wool Sorters' Disease'.

Diagnosis
Cutaneous anthrax is distinguished from boils and carbuncles by the pain and tenderness which occur in the latter two conditions and by culture of *Staph. aureus* from the pus. Other diseases which may cause confusion include vaccinia cowpox in cattlemen and orf in sheep handlers; both conditions may be diagnosed rapidly by electron microscopy. Anthrax is diagnosed by the presence of large Gram-positive bacilli in direct smears from suspicious lesions, and by culture and identification of the organism. Bacteriological confirmation is not possible in every case, particularly if antibiotics have been given. Confirmation may then be obtained by a rising anthrax antibody titre in paired sera; a procedure available at the Microbiological Research Establishment, Porton, Wiltshire.

Prognosis
In untreated cutaneous anthrax there is a mortality of about 15 per cent due to complicating septicaemia, but this is considerably reduced by antibiotic therapy. The rare pulmonary and gastrointestinal forms are usually fatal.

Treatment
The organism is highly sensitive to penicillin and this is the drug of choice, given intramuscularly in doses of the order of 3–4 mega units/day in divided doses. The organism is also sensitive to tetracycline and chloramphenicol, either of which is used in a patient who is allergic to penicillin. Local antibiotic treatment is unnecessary.

Prevention
Animals suspected of having anthrax are killed and cremated, or buried deeply in lime. A post-mortem is not allowed. Animals found dead from this disease are similarly disposed of. The Medical Officer of Environmental Health is notified of all human and animal cases and in addition anthrax in an industrial worker is notifiable to HM Chief Inspector of Factories. Human and animal contacts are kept under observation, and disinfection is carried out.

Many imported animal products such as wool and hair are disinfected at the port of entry. Workers handling potentially infective material such as hides are warned to report all suspicious skin lesions. Protective clothing and care of skin cuts is important, and dust extraction is necessary in some industries.

An effective vaccine is available from the Public Health Laboratory, and is given to workers who may be exposed to anthrax by their occupation. Four intramuscular injections of 0·5 ml are given with intervals of three weeks between the first, second and third doses and an interval of six months between the third and fourth doses. Booster doses of 0·5 ml at yearly intervals are advised. Reactions are uncommon. The use of this vaccine in recent years has greatly reduced the incidence of anthrax in high-risk industries.

CHAPTER 34

Leptospirosis

Organisms of the group *Leptospira* produce a febrile illness in man and animals throughout the world. In Britain three types of infection predominate and in the last eight years there have been 171 diagnosed cases with 31 deaths (averaging 20 cases per year with four deaths). Most of the cases were due to *L. icterohaemorrhagiae* with smaller numbers due to *L. canicola* and *L. hebdomadis*. In the more severe cases there are signs of renal, hepatic and meningeal involvement.

Epidemiology

(*a*) *Weil's disease*
Weil first described the disease in Germany in 1886, and the causative organism *L. icterohaemorrhagiae* was isolated in Japan in 1915. The organism commonly infects rats, but dogs, cattle and pigs are susceptible. In most animals, infection is established in the kidney, and the organism is excreted in the

urine. If the organism reaches fresh water, it can survive for more than a month, although it rapidly dies in dry conditions. Leptospirae gain entry to human hosts via skin abrasions or a mucous membrane. In Britain, Weil's Disease is largely an occupational hazard among farmers, sewage workers, fish workers and coal miners. Cases also arise from bathing in polluted water. No age is immune, but most cases occur in adults. Cases occur throughout the year. The severity of the disease varies greatly, and undoubtedly many non-jaundiced cases are not diagnosed. Although jaundice is not the cause of death, it is a good index of severity, since most fatalities occur in those who are jaundiced.

(b) Canicola fever

This disease was only recognized in Britain in 1955. *L. canicola*, the causative organism, is a common cause of disease in dogs and pigs. In dogs, the infection causes a nephritis, which may pass unnoticed, and many excrete the organism for months after recovery. Between 25 per cent and 50 per cent of dogs show serological evidence of infection. The disease occurs more commonly in domestic rather than occupational circumstances, occasional cases having nursed a sick dog, but outbreaks in pig farms have been reported. Bathing in fresh water polluted by dogs' urine is an occasional cause of the disease. All age groups are susceptible, but as with Weil's Disease, most cases occur in adults. Cases occur throughout the year, with an increased incidence in the autumn. Canicola fever is not usually a severe disease.

(c) Hebdomadis infection

Cases have been reported mainly from Scotland and South West England, and are mostly in farmers. Reservoirs of infection include field mice and voles from which cattle may be infected.

Pathology

The illness begins with bloodstream invasion, followed by localization in many organs. In the liver, there is a hepatitis producing jaundice. In the heart there is myocarditis producing circulatory failure. In the kidney there is an acute nephritis with a tendency to tubular necrosis and acute renal failure. In the nervous system there is involvement of the meninges, producing a non-suppurative meningitis. Microscopically there is an acute inflammatory reaction, particularly affecting capillary vessels which show bleeding.

Incubation period
This is commonly about 10 days with limits of 5–19 days.

Clinical picture
(*a*) *Weil's disease*
In most cases the onset is abrupt with high fever, profuse sweating and severe headache, the patient soon becoming prostrate. There is usually conjunctival suffusion, and pain and tenderness of the muscles of the back and limbs. Most cases show evidence of nephritis with protein, red and white cells and casts in the urine. The more severe cases show oliguria, progressing in some to acute anuric renal failure.

About half the cases show evidence of a haemorrhagic tendency with petechial rash, epistaxis, haematuria, and occasionally gastrointestinal bleeding. A similar number show meningeal irritation with neck and spinal rigidity and an abnormal CSF. The more severe cases develop jaundice about the 5th day of illness, and this will continue to deepen for a week or more. The illness tends to be at its worst about the 14th day, and most of the fatalities occur around this time. Death is usually due to acute renal failure or to circulatory failure caused by the myocarditis.

Improvement starts in the 3rd week; the pyrexia subsides, jaundice fades and the urinary output improves, often with a diuretic phase. The patient requires a protracted convalescence before returning to normal activity, but recovery is eventually complete. Milder cases do occur, without the development of jaundice or acute renal failure, when the illness is shorter and without fatality. In a minority of the cases, there is a relapse of the jaundice.

(*b*) *Canicola fever and hebdomadis infection*
The clinical illness is much milder than Weil's Disease. The majority of cases show only a febrile lymphocytic meningitis and evidence of nephritis or hepatitis is unusual. Cases may only be distinguished from viral meningitis by occupational exposure and by serology.

Diagnosis

In the early febrile stage, the diagnosis may be impossible although occupational exposure, the severe muscle pain and conjunctival suffusion may be suggestive. In the later stages, the combination of jaundice and renal damage should lead to a provisional diagnosis, as few other conditions, apart from certain types of chemical poisoning and collagen diseases, will produce these. The diagnosis can be confirmed by a rising antibody titre. This will distinguish the type of infection, and will be positive after the first week of illness. Although the organism can be isolated from the blood or urine by animal inoculation, this is a dangerous procedure, not usually undertaken by routine laboratories. Blood counts show a polymorph leucocytosis. When signs of meningitis are present the CSF, although clear, will show a raised protein and lymphocytic pleocytosis, with a normal sugar.

Prognosis

The mortality in jaundiced cases of Weil's Disease is about 15 per cent. It is not yet known whether the availability of haemodialysis for cases in acute renal failure has improved the mortality.

Treatment

Although penicillin and tetracycline are fully effective in preventing leptospiral infection in laboratory animal experiments, the drugs appear to do very little in the established disease. There is a good case for giving tetracycline to a patient at the very onset of suggestive symptoms when a suspicious occupational history is known. In the event of acute renal failure, the usual fluid-restricted, salt-free, high-calorie regime is necessary. If, in spite of this, diuresis does not occur, and the blood urea and serum potassium reach dangerous levels, haemodialysis will be necessary.

Prevention

Workers at risk should be equipped with rubber boots and protective clothing, and adequate washing facilities should be provided. They should be informed of the importance of reporting minor wounds and abrasions. Measures to destroy rat and mice populations are worthwhile. Publicity is necessary as regards the danger of bathing in stagnant pools, and sluggish streams which are usually rat infested. Dogs should be vaccinated against leptospirosis, and pet owners should be made aware of the dangers of urine contamination, when nursing a sick dog.

CHAPTER 35

Clostridial Infections

The clostridia are a large group of anaerobic bacteria which normally inhabit the gut of animal species and also of man. They are widely distributed in soil and dust, where they survive for very long periods due to the formation of spores which are resistant to heat and to drying. They are capable of causing a variety of diseases in man, usually by the elaboration of exotoxins.

1 Gas gangrene

Clostridia are common in wound infections, where, in normal aerobic conditions, they are incapable of growth and are of little significance. However, in wounds which contain necrotic and avascular tissue, they may multiply and produce toxins which cause necrosis of surrounding muscle and other soft tissues, with the production of gas locally, together with a very severe systemic upset. The most important organisms are *Cl. welchii* (*Cl. perfringens*), *Cl. septicum* and *Cl. oedematiens*, and infections are often caused by a combination of types. The usual portal of entry is a penetrating or lacerated wound particularly if a foreign body, clothing or soil are present. Other sites may be an intramuscular injection (particularly when preparations containing adrenaline are used), a surgical wound or the post partum uterus. In surgical practice, gas gangrene most frequently follows mid-thigh amputations, the source of infection being the bowel of the patient. Occasional small outbreaks in surgical units have been traced to persistent contamination of operating theatres. After an incubation period of 1–6 days, the area surrounding the wound rapidly becomes gangrenous, the skin blackens and the muscles turn grey and become friable. There is usually a dark-coloured, highly offensive discharge. The tissues surrounding the necrotic area become oedematous, discoloured and crepitant with gas, and gangrenous changes may extend rapidly. The patient is severely ill with fever, tachycardia and hypotension, and may develop acute renal failure, or jaundice due to severe haemolysis.

Treatment
Surgical excision of the gangrenous area should be carried out whenever possible. Hyperbaric oxygen treatment will limit the spread of infection and may reclaim borderline areas; this may be of considerable value both before and after surgery. The organisms are sensitive to penicillin, but its use is only an adjunct to surgical and hyperbaric oxygen treatment. A polyvalent antitoxin is available but is of very doubtful value and may cause severe general reactions. In cases of severe haemolysis, exchange transfusion has been recommended.

Prevention
In accident cases, thorough surgical toilet of wounds, followed by a full course of penicillin are the most effective measures. The risk of gas gangrene following mid-thigh amputation is such that it is recommended that all cases have prophylactic penicillin. If a local outbreak occurs in a surgical unit, investigation must include the operating theatre and its ventilation system.

2 'Clostridium perfringens (welchii)' gastroenteritis

Heat-resistant strains of Type A *Cl. perfringens* produce toxin which is capable of causing foodborne outbreaks of gastroenteritis, particularly in the elderly. The source of infection is usually directly from the gut of a carcase of an animal or chicken, and infection may be conveyed from kitchen dust or contaminated hands. The vehicle of infection is usually made-up meat or chicken dishes which are cooked and allowed to cool, before being eaten the following day either cold or inadequately reheated.

Clinical picture

After an incubation period of about 12 hours (limits 2–24 hours), there is an abrupt onset of colicky abdominal pain and diarrhoea. Vomiting and vertigo are occasional features. The illness is mild, often lasts less than 24 hours, and there is no mortality.

The diagnosis is established by the isolation of *Cl. welchii* from the faeces or vomit of cases and from food remains.

Prevention

Important measures are high standards of hygiene in the kitchen and the avoidance of bulk reheating of food in institutions.

3 Botulism

Cl. botulinum is common in the soil and may contaminate foodstuffs in which it may multiply in anaerobic conditions and produce a powerful neurotoxin. The disease is usually associated with the consumption of preserved or canned foods such as meat, fish, fruit and vegetables, which have been inadequately heat treated. It is very rare, only seven small outbreaks having been reported in Britain.

Clinical picture

After an incubation period of 12–36 hours, there is the onset of vomiting, tiredness, thirst and paralysis of muscles of the eye and of swallowing. Within 24 hours, flaccid paralysis of the limb and trunk muscles develops, leading to death from respiratory failure in half of the cases. The temperature is normal throughout. Recovery is gradual over a period of weeks or months, but is eventually complete.

The diagnosis is established by the demonstration in guineapigs of toxin in the blood or vomit. The isolation of *Cl. botulinum* from the faeces is not significant.

Treatment

Botulinus antitoxin is of doubtful value, and the main treatment is the maintenance of breathing by tracheotomy and artificial respiration.

Prevention
Modern and efficient commercial standards of canning prevent botulism; most of the outbreaks have been due to inadequate home preservation of food.

Infant botulism
It has been recognized recently that in the first few months of life, the spontaneous colonization of the gut by *Cl. botulinum* may produce sufficient toxin to cause illness. In most cases the illness is mild and transient with constipation and lethargy as prominent features, but in a few infants, the illness is more severe with difficulty in swallowing, paralytic squints and flaccid limb and trunk weakness.

The diagnosis is confirmed by the finding of botulinus toxin in faeces specimens. Spontaneous recovery is usual.

4 Tetanus

Cl. tetani from the soil may contaminate a wound where, under anaerobic conditions, it multiplies and produces the toxin which causes tetanus. This disease is characterized by hypertonicity of skeletal muscle with superimposed 'spasms' leading to respiratory distress.

Epidemiology
The causative organism, *Cl. tetani*, is present in the bowel of many herbivorous animals, especially the horse, so that pasture-land becomes contaminated and, under aerobic conditions, the organism forms spores which persist almost indefinitely. The spores are resistant to boiling and to many chemical disinfectants. They may gain entry to a wound which has been contaminated by soil, and will multiply if necrotic tissue is present there. The portal of entry is normally a wound, but it may be a chronic leg ulcer, chronic otitis media or rarely a surgical incision. In tropical countries neonatal tetanus is common, because of the practice of covering the umbilical stump with dung or mud. The disease most commonly affects people in active outdoor occupations, and high risk groups include farmers, gardeners, military personnel, field sportsmen and cotton workers. Tetanus is now less common in children because of routine active immunization during infancy, but has apparently

become more common in the elderly in recent years. The disease only became notifiable in 1968 so that the incidence is not accurately known, but it is estimated that there are about 40–50 cases a year in England and Wales. The disease produces no immunity so that second attacks occasionally occur.

Incubation period
This is usually 5–15 days, but may be considerably longer in mild forms of the disease; incubation periods below 10 days tend to be associated with severe disease.

Clinical picture
The first symptom is usually trismus, a painful stiffening of the jaw muscles with difficulty in opening the mouth. The painful stiffness progresses in about 24 hours to affect the muscles of the neck, back, chest and abdominal wall. The arms and legs are only slightly affected. Within 1–3 days, intermittent spasmodic contractions of the stiffened muscles occur, causing great pain and distress to the patient, and are often accompanied by pallor and profuse sweating. These 'spasms' cause grimacing of the face, the 'risus sardonicus', and arching of the neck and back muscles, termed opisthotonus. More important is the contraction of the respiratory muscles which results in respiratory embarrassment, occasionally progressing to pallid cyanosis. The spasms may occur spontaneously, or may result from stimuli such as noise, voluntary movements or coughing; for this reason, the patient attempts to avoid movements and to suppress cough. The combination of respiratory muscle contraction and suppression of cough leads to progressive deterioration in respiratory function. In severe cases, signs of sympathetic nervous over-activity may appear, including profuse sweating, swinging pyrexia, intermittent or sustained large fluctuations in blood pressure, tachycardia, cardiac arrythmias and even cardiac arrest. In cases who survive, the spasms gradually diminish in number and severity after 2–3 weeks, and the muscle rigidity disappears in a further 1–2 weeks.

In mild cases there is often a prolonged incubation period and generalized muscular rigidity without spasms. A rare and very mild form of the disease causes only local rigidity near to the injury after a very long incubation period.

Diagnosis

The diagnosis is made on clinical grounds, but may be confirmed by the isolation of *Cl. tetani* from the wound. The organism is cultured under anaerobic conditions. When trismus is the presenting feature, tetanus must be distinguished from mumps and from an abscess associated with an impacted wisdom tooth.

Acute dystonic reactions from tranquillizer drugs such as phenothiazines and the anti-emetic drug metoclopramide are commonly confused with tetanus and the dramatic response to 2 mg intravenous benztropine is diagnostic in such cases. Tetanus must also be distinguished from classical strychnine poisoning.

Prognosis

The mortality of untreated severe tetanus is about 60 per cent, but this has been reduced by modern management to 10–20 per cent. The consequences of sympathetic nerve overactivity have become the main cause of death in specialized treatment centres. Mild or localized tetanus has no mortality.

Treatment

Tetanus is treated in specially equipped designated centres.

1 The wound is surgically excised as early as possible.

2 Penicillin is given for 10 days, to eradicate persisting foci of *Cl. tetani*.

3 Human antitetanus immunoglobulin is given in a dose of 1000–2000 mg. The product is completely safe but probably does not play an important role in the management of the established disease.

4 If spasms are not occurring, intramuscular chlorpromazine or promazine (adult dose 100 mg 6-hourly) is given to sedate and relax the patient.

If spasms are already present or if they develop, tracheotomy is carried out and a cuffed tube is inserted. If the spasms are severe enough to cause sweating, pallor or cyanosis, the patient is immediately paralysed with curare, and respiration is maintained by an intermittent positive-pressure respirator. Curare is continued for two to three weeks in a dose sufficient to keep the patient completely relaxed (adult dose 15–30 mg every hour intravenously or intramuscularly with hyalase) and is only discontinued when trial periods without the drug show that spasms are no longer occurring. During the period of artificial respiration, intensive chest physiotherapy and regular aspiration of secretions are necessary to prevent infection and atelectasis. In spite of this, infections with *Pseudomonas sp.* and *Staph. aureus* are common and require additional antibiotic therapy. *Pseudomonas sp.* infection is treated with gentamicin, colistin or carbenicillin. Signs of sympathetic overactivity are treated with 'blocking' drugs, suchas practolol and bethanidine used in combination. Tube feeding, bladder catheterization and care of the skin are important.

5.   Tetanus cases subsequently require active immunization, as the disease does not produce immunity.

Prevention
The main preventive measure is active immunization with tetanus toxoid, as part of the routine programme in children. The primary course is given in infancy, with a booster dose on school entry, and such a programme has been routine practice in most areas since triple antigen became available in 1956. Ideally, a 2nd booster dose is given on leaving school and a further dose when an injury is sustained. Active immunization is also given to selected groups of adults such as military personnel and nurses, and could be usefully extended to other high risk groups, such as farmers, gardeners and field sport players. In the last few years the uptake of tetanus vaccine in children has fallen to about 50 per cent nationally. Unless this is rectified, there will be an increase in the incidence of tetanus as these susceptible children grow older and more active.

Management of patients with wounds
Equine antitetanus serum (ATS) is no longer used. Surgical toilet and antibiotics alone are not reliable in the prevention of tetanus.
Modern recommendations are as follows:
1   In the previously adequately immunized patient, a dose of 0·5 ml adsorbed tetanus toxoid is given provided that one year has elapsed since the last booster injection.
2   In the previously unimmunized patients of all age groups, passive protection with human antitetanus immunoglobulin

(dose 250–500 mg) should be given in the following categories of trauma:

(i)   Wounds or burns sustained more than six hours before treatment.

(ii)   Wounds or burns sustained at any time with one or more of the following features.

(a)   significant devitalized tissue
(b)   puncture wounds
(c)   contamination with soil
(d)   containing foreign bodies
(e)   animal bites
(f)   clinical signs of infection

Otherwise passive protection is not required, the wound is treated surgically and penicillin or tetracycline is given if indicated. In addition for future protection, active immunization with adsorbed tetanus toxoid (ATT) should be started and adequate arrangements made for completion of the course.

CHAPTER 36

Malaria and Toxoplasmosis

1   Malaria

Epidemiology

Malaria is the most common and serious of all tropical infections and is endemic throughout most of Asia and the Pacific, South and Central America and Africa and the Middle East. The infection is caused by protozoal parasites of the Plasmodium family. *Plasmodium vivax, ovale* and *malariae* cause a benign relapsing disease and are the most common varieties in Asia and America. *Plasmodium vivax* malaria importations into Britain have greatly increased in recent years due to a serious recrudescence of the disease in India and Pakistan. *Plasmodium falciparum* causes a more serious or fatal disease which is very common in tropical Africa but also occurs in other malarial zones.

The disease is transmitted by anopheline mosquito bite and both man and the mosquito act as reservoirs of infection.

In endemic regions, the local population commonly suffer from chronic malaria with anaemia and debility with an enlarged spleen. Because of partial immunity, acute episodes of fever seldom occur but the chronic disease proves a serious economic hindrance to the areas involved. Non-immune travellers to endemic areas develop acute febrile disease. More than a thousand cases of malaria are imported each year into Britain, but there is no spread of the disease in this country.

Clinical picture

(*a*) *Benign relapsing malaria (P. vivax, ovale and malariae)*
Following transmission by mosquito bite, a red blood cell cycle of infection develops causing an acute febrile illness. At the same time a persistent reservoir of infection develops in the liver and reticulo-endothelial system which is responsible for later relapses of the disease.

The disease presents abruptly with fever, rigors and malaise, on alternate days with *P. vivax* and *ovale* infections, or every third day with the rarer *P. malariae* infection. The spleen is frequently enlarged. The diagnosis is confirmed by the demonstration of parasites at varying stages of development in blood films. After the primary infection, similar febrile episodes may recur for 2–3 years with *P. vivax* infection and for 20 years or even longer with *P. malariae* infections. In the case of a patient taking regular prophylactic drugs in the tropics, the first attack might occur several months after returning to Britain.

(*b*) *Malignant malaria (P. falciparum)*
P. falciparum is the main cause of malaria in tropical Africa, but does occur in other malarial regions, particularly in South East Asia. After transmission by mosquito bite, a severe red blood cell cycle of infection develops within a month. There is no persisting reservoir of infection in the liver so that relapses do not occur. In the red cells there is rapid multiplication of the parasite and this is responsible for the serious nature of the disease. The onset is abrupt and the fever is usually persistent

and irregular, only occasionally showing a tertian pattern; the spleen is commonly enlarged. The large numbers of damaged infected red cells may cause serious damage to the capillary circulation causing ischaemia, particularly in the brain, the kidneys, the myocardium and the gut. This may lead to the abrupt development of an encephalopathy (cerebral malaria) with mental confusion, convulsions and coma which may be fatal. Otherwise there may be acute renal failure, mycocarditis with peripheral circulatory failure or severe watery diarrhoea.

The diagnosis is confirmed by the demonstration of uniform small-ring parasites in blood films.

Treatment

1   Benign relapsing malaria (P. vivax)

Chloroquine or amodiaquine is the initial drug of choice, given for three days. To eliminate the hepatic reservoir of infection and prevent relapses a further 14-day course of primaquine is necessary. (For dosage see Table 9). Primaquine may cause severe haemolysis particularly in patients deficient in the enzyme glucose-6-phosphate dehydrogenase (G6PD).

2   Malignant malaria (P. falciparum)

Chloroquine or amodiaquine in a three-day course is curative. In a severe illness intramuscular chloroquine is preferred and corticosteroids are reported to be of benefit in cerebral malaria. (See Table 9 for dosage).

3   Resistant malaria

In several areas, particularly where antimalarial drugs have been used extensively such as Indo-China and South-East Asia, drug resistant falciparum parasites are common (drug resistance has not been a problem in Africa). Such infections may be treated with quinine by slow intravenous infusion.

In any fulminating episode of *falciparum* malaria from Asia there is a case for adding quinine to the therapy because of the possibility of resistance.

Prevention

The eradication of malaria by drainage schemes and insecticides has been successful in many islands, including Cyprus, Singapore, Hong Kong and the Caribbean, and in a few

TABLE 9

Drug	Alternative name	Prophylaxis dose (adult)	Treatment dose (adult)	Comments
Chloroquine (base)	Avloclor, Nivaquine	300 mg once weekly	600 mg stat 300 mg in 6 hours 300 mg 2nd and 3rd days	These two drugs are the first choice in treatment and the last choice in prophylaxis
Amodiaquine (base)	Camoquin	400 mg once weekly	600 mg stat 400 mg 2nd and 3rd days	
Proguanil	Paludrine	100 mg daily	—	These two drugs are the first choice in prophylaxis and are not used in treatment
Pyrimethamine	Daraprim	25 mg once weekly	—	
Primaquine	—	—	7·5 mg TDS for 14 days	To prevent relapse in *vivax* malaria
Quinine dihydrochloride solution	—	—	650 mg in 500 ml saline, 2 or 3 times in 24 hours intravenously	Treatment of resistant or very severe *falciparum* malaria
Chloroquine phosphate solution	—	—	300 mg of 5 % solution (40 mg/ml) twice in 24 hours intramuscularly	

developed mainland countries including Israel, Lebanon and South Africa.

In existing malarial zones, personal precautions including insect-repellent creams and mosquito nets are still worthwhile but the main measure is the prophylactic use of drugs. These drugs must be started one day before entering a malarial zone and continued for one month after leaving. Proguanil or pyrimethamine are the drugs of choice, being both effective and little used in treatment. If local parasite resistance to these drugs is found, then chloroquine may be used as a prophylactic although this will favour eventual drug resistance. Chloroquine should not be used for very long-term prophylaxis because of the risk of cumulative optic nerve damage.

In hyperendemic malarial zones, especially West Africa, the prophylactic dose of proguanil (Paludrine) or pyrimethamine (Daraprim) may be doubled. (See Table 9 for dosage.) Maloprin (Daraprim and dapsone) taken once weekly is a suitable alternative.

The Malaria Reference Laboratory and the World Health Organization Malaria Reference Centre is at the London School of Hygiene and Tropical Medicine.

2 Toxoplasmosis

This is caused by the protozoan parasite *Toxoplasma gondii*, which is found in many animals and birds, and may be spread to man by contact with animals, particularly the domestic cat. Several hundred cases are diagnosed each year in Britain, about half the cases being in infancy with predominantly ocular disease, and most of the remainder in adults with pyrexial illness.

(a) *Congenital toxoplasmosis*

Infection in pregnant women may affect the fetus by way of the placenta. Congenital infection is mainly characterized by a choroidoretinitis. This may be accompanied by a diffuse encephalitis with a raised protein level and lymphocyte count in the CSF. The mortality of encephalitis is about 10 per cent but many of the survivors show sequelae such as impaired vision, intracranial calcification, hydrocephalus and mental retardation. The fetus in subsequent pregnancies is not affected.

(*b*) *Acquired toxoplasmosis*

This occurs in adults and presents with low-grade fever, tiredness and lymphadenopathy persisting for several weeks. There have also been rare instances of fatal acquired encephalitis.

The diagnosis is confirmed by a complex but sensitive antibody detection dye test, only carried out in certain Public Health Laboratories.

The recommended treatments are either a combination of sulphonamide (adult dose 3 g daily) and pyrimethamine (adult dose 25 mg daily) or the antibiotic spiramycin (adult dose 2 g daily). These treatments are beneficial in (i) reducing the incidence of fetal defects when given to the infected pregnant woman; (ii) improving ocular disease when combined with corticosteroids; and (iii) controlling fever and symptoms in adult syndromes.

CHAPTER 37

Intestinal Worm Infections

There are many thousands of varieties of parasitic worms, infesting all forms of animal and plant life, but only a few types are of importance to man. Worm infections in man usually result either from inadequate sanitary conditions where soil or vegetable crops are contaminated with faeces or from the eating of uncooked animal flesh. In developed countries only the threadworm flourishes because of its simple bowel–hand–mouth method of spread. In their passage through the human host worms often adopt a complicated route sometimes referred to as 'round-the-houses'. Generally, worms habituated to the human host complete their cycle without provoking much tissue reaction, whereas worms habituated to another animal species provoke a severe tissue reaction in man. In Britain a variety of round- and tape-worm infections are diagnosed, although the infection usually originates in tropical countries. In many of these imported cases multiple infections are found. The diagnosis is usually reached by the finding of worms or their eggs (ova) in the faeces. Many worm infections provoke a striking eosinophilia of 10–50 per cent.

NEMATODES (Roundworms)

1 Threadworm (*Enterobius vermicularis*)

This is the commonest worm infection in Britain with a prevalence as high as 20 per cent in some studies. Usually several members of a household or institution are affected. Threadworm is most common in children and may persist with relapses and remissions for months or years.

Cycle of infection

Adult worms are present in the colon and rectum from where the gravid female emerges at night to deposit eggs in the perianal skin. These eggs are then carried by hands, clothing or dust to be ingested by the same person or by new hosts. The eggs pass down the intestine maturing slowly to larvae and adult worms which fix to the colon wall and breed there. The cycle is complete in about a month.

Clinical picture

When the eggs are deposited, pronounced perianal itching may occur, which is worst at night. The white, slightly motile, gravid female thread-like worms may be visible in the faeces. The infection is otherwise asymptomatic, even if its presence may cause some anxiety to the family. There is very slender evidence linking thread worm infections with appendicitis or allergic asthma.

Diagnosis

This is made by the appearance of visible worms and the perianal itching. It may be confirmed by the application of Scotch tape to the perianal skin, preferably in the early morning. The tape is then applied to a glass slide and the ova are seen under low-power microscopy.

Treatment
It is important to treat the whole family or group at one time. The house is thoroughly cleaned to remove eggs from toilets, floors and dust. Clothing and bedding are changed and laundered. Personal bathing eliminates ova from the skin.

Piperazine is the drug of choice. It may be given either in a large single dose mixed with senna, repeated two weeks later, or as the elixir in a seven-day course. The drug is safe but is not given if renal impairment or poorly controlled epilepsy is present. An alternative effective drug is viprynium given in a single dose repeated in two weeks; this drug stains the stools red. (See Table 10 for dosage.)

2 (a) Human roundworm (*Ascaris lumbricoides*)

This infection is very common in underdeveloped countries and is found occasionally in rural areas of this country. Most cases occur in children.

Cycle of infection
Eggs are ingested either directly from uncooked contaminated vegetable foods, or indirectly from hands contaminated by soil, door handles or toilet fittings. In the upper intestine the eggs develop into larvae about 1 mm in length. These penetrate the gut wall and proceed, via the bloodstream, to the liver and then to the lungs. In the lungs they enter the alveoli and ascend the bronchi and trachea to the pharynx and are swallowed into the intestine where they develop into large pale pink adult roundworms, 20–30 cm in length. The adult worms move slowly against peristalsis in the bowel where they breed and produce large numbers of eggs which are passed into the soil in the faeces, completing the cycle.

Clinical picture
Many infections are completely asymptomatic, although the passage of an adult worm may occasion the patient lasting anxiety and distress. Larval worms in the liver may cause inflammatory changes with tender hepatomegaly. Larvae in the lungs may cause an allergic pneumonitis with wheezing dyspnoea, X-ray infiltration and an intense blood eosinophilia.

Adult worms in the bowel may cause abdominal pain or

TABLE 10

Treatment of nematode infestations

Drug	Proprietary preparations	Adult dose	Children's dose	Effective in:	Notes
Piperazine	Pripsen sachets (Piperazine 4 g + senna)	1 sachet (repeated in 2 weeks)	Aged 3–10 years $\frac{2}{3}$ sachet (repeated in 2 weeks)	Threadworm Roundworm	Dizziness and ataxia
	Elixir Antepar (750 mg/5 ml)	15–30 ml daily for 7 days	6–12 years 10–15 ml 1–4 years 5 ml under 1 year 2·5 ml daily for 7 days	Threadworm Roundworm	
Viprynium	Vanquin (50 mg tablets 50 mg/5 ml suspension)	5–10 mg/kg single dose (repeated in 2 weeks)	5–10 mg/kg single dose (repeated in 2 weeks)	Threadworm	Stains stools red
Bephenium granules	Alcopar (5 g packets)	5–10 g single dose daily for 2–3 days	1 g per year of life single dose daily for 2–3 days	Hookworm Roundworm	
Tetrachlorethylene	Capsules BP	1–3 ml single dose (repeated in 2 weeks)	0·1 ml/kg single dose (repeated in 2 weeks)	Hookworm	More toxic. More effective against *Necator*

Thiabendazole	Mintezol (500-mg tablets)	50 mg/kg daily for 2–3 days	50 mg/kg daily for 2–3 days	Hookworm Strongyloidiasis Trichiniasis Whip worm Cutaneous larva migrans	Nausea, drowsiness, vertigo
Mebendazole	Vermox (100 mg tablets)	100 mg bd for 3 days	2–6 years 50 mg bd for 3 days	Hookworm Whipworm	Poorly absorbed
Hexylresorcinol	Crystoids antihelminthic	1 g single dose	0·1 g per year of life single dose	Roundworm Hookworm Whip worm	Starvation on day of treatment
Diethylcarbamazine	Hetrazan Banocide	10 mg/kg daily for 3 weeks	10 mg/kg daily for 3 weeks	Toxocariasis	

allergic urticarial rashes. Occasionally heavy infestations may result in intestinal obstruction or other mechanical disorders such as bile duct obstruction.

Diagnosis
This is made by the passage of adult worms or the finding of ova in faecal smears or concentrates. Eosinophilia in the blood occurs at the larval migration stage but lessens as the adult stage is reached.

Treatment
Piperazine is the drug of choice and is usually effective. Bephenium (Alcopar) is a safe alternative. Hexylresorcinol is another safe and effective alternative, but is irritant to the mouth and the patient must be starved on the day of administration (see Table 10 for dosage). In Britain roundworm is readily controlled but in tropical countries reinfection usually occurs.

2 (b) Animal roundworm (*Toxocara canis* and *T. cati*)

These are roundworms normally occurring in dogs and cats. *T. canis* is most often found in puppies and pregnant bitches, and the ova will widely contaminate the soil. These ova may be ingested by children and in rare instances may lead to an invasive condition, one of the forms of visceral larva migrans. There is a larval infiltration with eosinophilic inflammation of many organs including the liver, lungs, skin, eyes and nervous system.

Clinically there may be hepatic enlargement, skin rashes, choroiditis, retinitis and chest X-ray infiltration. Eye involvement may lead to permanent visual impairment.

The diagnosis is suggested by the clinical features with the finding of eosinophilia and hypergammaglobulinaemia and is confirmed by specific skin and serology tests.

Treatment is largely supportive but larval worms can be killed by diethylcarbamazine (see Table 10 for dosage).

3 (a) Human hookworm

The main varieties are *Ancylostoma duodenale* (common hookworm) and *Necator americanus* ('the American killer'). Infection is common in all tropical and subtropical countries where sewage disposal is inadequate and where people walk barefoot.

Cycle of infection

Infected faeces containing eggs are passed on to the soil where the larval stage develops. These may then penetrate the intact skin of the bare foot and pass via the lymphatics into the bloodstream. The larvae are finally trapped in the lungs where they pass to the alveoli, bronchi and pharynx when they are swallowed and fix to the wall of the upper intestine, growing to the adult size of about 1 cm. Egg production then takes place completing the cycle.

Clinical picture

At the time of infection, there may be itching skin lesions at the site of entry, known as 'ground itch'. During larval migration there is an intense eosinophilia and may be an allergic pneumonitis.

The adult worms feed by sucking blood from the intestinal mucosa and in a heavy infection (more than 500 worms) a progressive and severe iron-deficiency and blood-loss anaemia will develop. Light infections (less than 50 worms) usually do not cause anaemia.

Diagnosis

This is made by the finding of ova in faecal smears or concentrates. The fall in haemoglobin reflects the heaviness of the infestation.

Treatment

Bephenium (Alcopar) is the drug of choice in hookworm infections. It may cure the infestation or at least will destroy the majority of the worms. Alternative drugs which may be used are thiabendazole, mebendazole, hexylresorcinol and tetrachlorethylene (see Table 10 for dosage). Treatment is satisfactory in a patient who has moved to Britain, but in tropical countries treatment is usually only temporarily successful because of reinfection. Anaemia responds to iron, but if very severe may require slow blood transfusion.

3 (b) Animal hookworm

Ancylostoma braziliense is a hookworm normally found in dogs and cats. Occasionally the larvae of this worm, present in the soil, may penetrate human skin and enter the cutaneous lymphatics. There is a fierce tissue reaction which shows as a slowly advancing serpiginous inflamed track on the skin of the lower limb. This is the commonest form of cutaneous larva migrans or 'creeping eruption'. The condition is self-limiting but may be aborted by freezing with carbon dioxide 'snow' on the active end of the track or by thiabendazole.

4 Trichiniasis

Originally an unimportant parasite of cannibalistic rats, the small roundworm *Trichinella spiralis* became established on a large scale in swill-fed pigs. In the pig the larvae invade the muscles. The cycle is maintained by the commercial feeding of pigs with swill which contains infected raw pork scraps. Man becomes involved by the ingestion of infected pork, usually as raw or undercooked sausage either eaten in that form or used as a cheap sandwich spread. In the human intestinal mucosa, ingested larvae mature to adult forms, producing ova which mature to larvae and then enter the bloodstream invading many organs. In striated muscle the larvae become permanently encysted, but in other tissues an eosinophilic inflammatory response occurs and the larvae are destroyed. The disease is common in America but there have only been a few outbreaks in Britain in recent decades.

Clinical picture

When the worms invade the intestinal mucosa there may be abdominal pain and diarrhoea. In the larval invasion stage, there is a systemic upset with sustained fever, periorbital oedema and pain in muscles and joints. In severe cases, there may be an allergic pneumonitis, myocarditis with failing blood pressure or neurological involvement leading to coma; some of these cases end fatally.

The acute illness settles over a period of weeks and slow recovery follows. The visceral worms are absorbed and the encysted worms in muscle calcify over a period of several years.

Diagnosis
There is an intense eosinophilia in the acute stages and from the third week of illness serology tests will become positive. Muscle biopsy will show the encysted worms, often in considerable numbers.

Treatment and prevention
Treatment is not satisfactory but corticosteroids may improve the acute systemic upset and thiabendazole may hasten the death of the larvae. It may be possible to reduce the infection by the heat treatment of pigswill. Inspection of pork at slaughterhouses often fails to identify infested carcases. The final link in the chain of infection is broken by adequate cooking of all pork products.

5 Whipworm (*Trichuris trichiura*)

This is a small roundworm occurring in all warm countries with poor sanitary facilities. The cycle of infection is a simple transfer of ova by the bowel–soil–hand–mouth route. Light infections are symptomless and harmless. Rarely a heavy infestation will cause abdominal pain, blood-streaked diarrhoea and anaemia. The diagnosis is made by the finding of eosinophilia in the blood and ova in the faeces. The treatments of choice are thiabendazole, mebendazole or hexylresorcinol.

6 Strongyloides stercoralis

This small roundworm is found in all tropical and subtropical countries where the whole life cycle may be 'free-living' in the soil. The cycle of infection in man may be similar to that of hookworm but in addition, ova produced in the bowel may mature to larvae which cause an autoinfection cycle, so that all cases should be treated. Many cases are asymptomatic but in some cases larvae may penetrate the skin around the anus, producing urticarial skin eruptions (larva currens) which tend to extend rapidly over the thighs and trunk. A heavy infestation may produce diarrhoea and anaemia. Thiabendazole is the treatment of choice.

TAPEWORMS (Cestodes)

Tapeworms are elongated flatworms which may reach 10 metres in length. They are hermaphrodite so that a single adult worm produces huge numbers of fertile eggs. Tapeworm infections behave in different ways in different vertebrate hosts:

(i) The intermediate host ingests ova which develop into larvae with invasion of the host animal's muscles and other organs.

(ii) The definitive host acquires the infection by the ingestion of the raw flesh of an intermediate host. In the definitive host, one or more adult worms develop in the gut where the head attaches to the upper intestine. The body of the worm consists largely of multiple flat egg-bearing segments which detach from time to time and may be seen in the faeces. The ova and segments in the faeces infect new intermediate hosts, completing the double cycle of infection.

Man is the definitive host to several varieties of tapeworm which are diagnosed by the identification of eggs or segments in the faeces. More seriously man may be the intermediate host with some varieties of tapeworm. A moderate eosinophilia of 10–25 per cent may occur in any tapeworm infection.

A HUMAN DEFINITIVE HOST INFECTIONS

1 Fish tapeworm (*Diphyllobothrium latum*) 5–10 m length

Man acquires infection with the fish tapeworm by the ingestion of raw freshwater fish. The infection is common in Scandinavia and the Far East, but is not found in Britain. The infection is usually with a single worm and is generally symptomless, but may cause vague intestinal symptoms. If the worm fixes at the upper end of the jejunum it may successfully compete for the host's dietary vitamin B12 and a megaloblastic anaemia may occur. Larva in untreated human sewage passed into rivers or lakes enters the fish feeding cycle and completes the cycle of infection possibly spreading the disease to neighbouring waters. The diagnosis is made by the finding of ova in the faeces.

2   Dwarf tapeworm (*Hymenolepis nana*)
1–2 cm length

This tapeworm is common in cats and may pass to man via the cat flea or from cat faeces. Alternatively infection may pass from man to man in a simple bowel–hand–mouth cycle. Man is a definitive host and commonly several members of a family are affected. The infection is usually symptomless but may cause vague abdominal symptoms or rarely diarrhoea. The diagnosis is made by the finding of characteristic double-walled ova in the faeces.

3   Beef tapeworm (*Taenia saginate*)
5–10 m length

Man is the only definitive host and acquires the infection by eating the undercooked flesh of the cow, the common intermediate host. The infection is usually symptomless but may cause great anxiety to the patient as the detached whitish-yellow opaque segments are motile and may emerge spontaneously from the anus. Infection in Britain is uncommon but is common in tropical countries. Infected carcases may be detected in slaughterhouses by examination of the masseter muscles.

4   Pork tapeworm (*Taenia solium*)
2–5 m length

Man is the only definitive host and acquires the infection by eating undercooked 'measly' pork or raw pork sausage. The adult worm infection usually causes no symptoms other than vague abdominal complaints. The diagnosis is made by the finding of white translucent segments in the faeces. More seriously man may also act as an intermediate host to *T. solium* causing cysticercosis (see below).

Treatment
All intestinal tapeworms are readily destroyed by niclosamide

H

(Yomesan) or dichlorophen (Antiphen). Occasionally the worms are not eradicated, ova or segments reappear in the faeces and retreatment is necessary. The dosage is as follows:

| | Adult | Children | | |
		6–12 years	1–5 years	Under 1 year
Niclosamide	1 g repeated in 1 hour before breakfast	0·5–1 g repeated in 1 hour	0·5 g single dose	250 mg single dose
Dichlorophen	6 g daily in divided doses for 2 days	1–2 g daily for 2 days	0·25–1 g daily for 2 days	

Prevention

Measures include (i) treatment of human cases, (ii) treatment of raw sewage, (iii) inspection of meat and pork in slaughterhouses, (iv) adequate cooking of fish, beef and pork, (v) deep-freezing which kills the larval worms.

B   HUMAN INTERMEDIATE HOST INFECTIONS

1   Cysticercosis (*Taenia solium*)

Man may be infected as an intermediate host either by the ingestion of food or water contaminated by ova from another human host or from ova produced by his own tapeworm in the intestine. The ova develop into larvae which penetrate the gut wall and invade the tissues, particularly skeletal muscle and the brain where they mature to cysticercus forms. During the invasive stage there may be slight fever, muscle aching and eosinophilia. After a latent period of several years the cysticercus forms die producing inflammatory and fibrotic lesions which eventually calcify. At this stage recurrent grand mal convulsions may occur or occasionally more diffuse neurological, ocular or mental disturbance.

The diagnosis is suspected in a patient who develops recurrent fits after living in the tropics for a period and may be confirmed by the finding of numerous fine calcified cysts on muscle X-ray and by serology tests. Treatment is usually symptomatic with anticonvulsant drugs, but occasionally may be by surgical removal of cysts from the eye or brain.

2 Hydatid cysts (*Echinococcus granulosus*)

The dog is the definitive host of this small tapeworm which produces large numbers of eggs in the faeces, contaminating grazing land and infecting sheep which are the usual intermediate host. The cycle is completed by the ingestion of infected raw sheep offal by dogs.

Man becomes an accidental intermediate host by close contact with dogs. The disease is particularly prevalent in the Middle East, but occurs in all sheep-rearing countries and has been reported in Wales. In man the ingested ova develop to embryo worms which penetrate the gut wall and invade the tissues. Most of these embryos are destroyed but one or more may survive and become encysted, usually in the liver, occasionally in the lung or rarely in other organs. These hydatid cysts gradually enlarge over a period of years, eventually reaching 5–20 cm in size. The fluid-filled cyst has a thick capsule and contains numerous infective protoscolices. Clinically the cysts present as a palpable slowly growing liver tumour or as a partially calcified circular lesion on chest X-ray. Large cysts in the liver may rupture spontaneously causing sudden pain, fever, allergic rashes and eosinophilia followed by the slow development of numerous daughter cysts throughout the peritoneal cavity. Large cysts in the lung may rupture causing an acute allergic pneumonitis with transformation of the cyst to a lung abscess. Smaller cysts may calcify gradually with the death of all living worm tissue.

The diagnosis is suggested by clinical or X-ray findings. Hepatic cysts may be demonstrated by liver scan or computerized axial tomography, and serological tests will provide confirmation.

Treatment
There have been isolated reports of slow resolution of cysts following treatment with the newer analogues of thiabendazole, particularly mebendazole in large doses. However, large cysts

of the liver or lung may need surgical removal to prevent the serious consequences of a spontaneous rupture. At operation cysts are first sterilized by the removal of cyst fluid and replacement with 10 per cent formalin to prevent contamination of the peritoneum or lung.

CHAPTER 38

Miscellaneous Infections

1 Orf

Orf or contagious pustular dermatitis is common in sheep and goats. It is caused by a virus which belongs to the pox virus group. Infection occasionally occurs in shepherds or abattoir workers, and presents as a single papular lesion, usually on the hand, forearm or face, which slowly develops to a large heaped-up multilocular painless vesicle with slight surrounding redness and induration. The lesion heals spontaneously in a few weeks, and there is no effective treatment. The diagnosis may be confirmed by the demonstration of the virus by electron microscopy.

2 Roseola infantum

This uncommon disease has been described as occurring in small epidemics in baby nurseries, mostly in the USA. While confirmation of the diagnosis is impossible, suspicious cases are reported from time to time in this country. It is thought to be of viral origin and occurs mainly in children under three years of age. After an incubation period of 5–15 days, there is pyrexia of 38–40°C which persists for 3–5 days with vomiting, irritability, restlessness and occasionally convulsions. As the temperature falls abruptly a discrete macular rash appears on the trunk. It spreads to the neck, face and proximal parts of the limbs, and usually persists for 1–2 days.

Diagnosis is made on clinical grounds. There is no recorded mortality and no effective treatment or preventive measures.

3   Winter vomiting disease

Outbreaks of this condition have been increasingly reported in recent years, particularly affecting families, schools and institutions. The cause is thought to be a virus, probably spread by droplet infection and in some outbreaks the Norwalk agent or other members of the parvovirus group or occasionally picornavirus types have been incriminated. The highest incidence occurs in the winter months. After an incubation period of 1–7 days, there is an abrupt onset of nausea with repeated vomiting. There may be headache, giddiness, abdominal discomfort or pain, mild diarrhoea and slight sore throat. Pyrexia if present is slight and transient. Symptoms usually resolve within 48 hours, and there is no mortality. The progression of an epidemic, by case-to-case spread over several days or weeks, distinguishes this conditions from food-borne gastroenteritis.

4   Candidosis

Candida (or *Monilia*) *albicans* is a saprophytic yeast present in the mouth and intestine of man, from which areas it is commonly isolated in the absence of significant infection.

The organisms may produce a superficial infection of the mucosa of the mouth, termed 'thrush', with the occurrence of multiple white plaques which may occasionally be wiped off. There is little local inflammatory reaction and no systemic upset. Thrush occurs in young babies or in adults suffering from debilitating disease.

Less common varieties of *Candida* infection are:

(a)   Low-grade vaginitis and perineal infection, often in diabetic or obese women.

(b)   Secondary infection in bronchiectatic or other chronically damaged lung tissue.

(c)   Generalized infection, spreading by the bloodstream in patients suffering from diseases such as leukaemia, lymphoma or collagen disease where the immunity mechanisms are disturbed. In such patients, normally innocuous yeasts or fungi may become invasive.

(d)   Muco-cutaneous candidiasis—this rare condition arises from a congenital fault in cell-mediated immunity. It presents with widespread persistent *Candida* infection of the skin and all mucous membranes.

The treatment of oral or vaginal thrush is by tropical Nystatin, or amphotericin B preparations. Respiratory infections may be improved by the inhalation of nystatin spray. Systemic infections are treated with intravenous infusions of amphotericin B in a daily dose increasing to 0·6 mg/kg body weight in a free-running five per cent dextrose drip. Toxic effects are very common and include nausea, vomiting, fever, thrombophlebitis, anaemia and renal damage. The newer drug 5-fluorocytosine is equally effective although a minority of candida strains are highly resistant. The drug is absorbed orally and is not toxic; the dosage is up to 200 mg/kg body weight per day.

A further new group of drugs, the imidazoles, is beginning to be used in both the topical and systemic fungal infections with promising results.

5   Stevens–Johnson syndrome

The aetiology of this condition is unknown; in some cases there is evidence of a mycoplasma or chlamydia infection, and in others a toxic reaction to drugs, such as sulphonamides, is suggested. The syndrome may be related to the milder condition of erythema multiforme; it occurs mainly in children and young adults and case-to-case spread is not seen. The disease varies widely in severity, and occasionally there are relapses at intervals of months or years.

The diagnostic clinical features are:

(a)   A prodromal period of fever and malaise, which lasts for one or more days.

(b)   A bright papular erythematous rash, confined to the face and limbs in mild cases, but generalized in severe cases. The papules vary in size and shape and 'target lesions' are common. In severe cases there is progression to vesicles and bullae with subsequent desquamation.

(c)   Ulcerative stomatitis.

(d)   Conjunctivitis.

(e)   Ulceration of the glans penis in a male, and of the female introitus.

(f)   Tendency to bronchitis or bronchopneumonia.

Among severe cases there is a mortality of about 10 per cent. The diagnosis depends on clinical recognition of the syndrome. Treatment by means of corticosteroids and broad spectrum antibiotics is recommended in severe cases, although there is little objective evidence that these measures influence the course of the disease.

6 Vincent's infection

Originally described as a specific disease, this is now considered to be a secondary infection of damaged tissue in the mouth or throat. The causes of such damage include viral infections, malnutrition, blood dyscrasias, operative or radiation trauma and the common gum disorders associated with dental disease. Spirochaetes and anaerobic organisms such as bacteroides, anaerobic cocci and fusobacteria are common secondary invaders. Necrotic mouth ulcers and occasionally gingival abscesses with offensive purulent discharge are characteristic features. These infections heal when the cause can be removed but may be improved by penicillin or metronidazole.

7 Listeriosis

Listeriosis is an infectious disease of animals and man caused by a Gram-positive bacillus called *Listeria monocytogenes.* The organisms are widespread in wild and domestic animals and birds throughout the world. Human infections are uncommon and during 1977, 47 cases were recorded in Britain, but the true incidence is probably more than this. It occurs in newborn infants when it apparently results from latent genital tract infection in the mother and is also encountered in adults, the majority of whom have a pre-existing disease such as cancer, chronic infection, autoimmune disease or who are otherwise immunosuppressed. The disease generally manifests itself either as meningitis or as speticaemia and the diagnosis is established by the isolation of the organisms from the CSF or blood. The treatment of choice is ampicillin given in large doses intravenously but the mortality is high (20–30 per cent).

8 Scabies

Scabies is an exclusively human skin infestation caused by the burrowing mite *Sarcoptes scabiei.* The mite flourishes in all climates including temperate and cold, and the incidence of the infestation appears to wax and wane in a country in roughly 10-year cycles.

Several members of a family or group are usually affected at the same time. Scabies spreads by close personal contact and it is rare for bedding or clothing to play a part in the spread. There are commonly only about 10 mites involved in a single case. The female mite after fertilization burrows into the epidermis, feeding on keratin, and deposits eggs which hatch into larvae and reach maturity in 2–3 weeks.

The majority of burrows are on the hands or forearms, particularly in the interdigital clefts of the fingers or the creases of the wrist, but occasionally burrows are found in the axillae, nipples, umbilicus, external genitalia or feet. The burrows appear as dark hair-like tracks in the skin sometimes punctuated by tiny vesicles and the entrance is often blocked by a plug of dirt. For several weeks the lesions are not irritant and are readily overlooked. After this time sensitization of the skin occurs often with the appearance of a scattered papular allergic rash accompanied by widespread severe itching which is worse at night or when the patient is warm. Scratching results in further skin trauma and the occurrence of secondarily infected superficial crusting. In the case of a reinfection with scabies the burrow sites begin to itch immediately.

The diagnosis is suggested by the degree of itching and the appearance of the rash and may be confirmed by the identification under low-power microscopy of a mite removed by needle-point from a burrow.

It is essential to treat all the members of a family or group simultaneously, preferably supervised by a community nurse. The patients have a warm soapy bath and are then completely coated, apart from the head, with 25 per cent benzyl benzoate emulsion which is allowed to dry on the skin. For successful treatment the application must be thorough and this is not usually possible when the patient attempts to apply his own treatment. The emulsion is not washed off and the application is repeated after two days, with a final bath the following day. Babies and young children particularly with secondarily infected lesions are often best treated in hospital. Equally effective and less irritant alternatives are 1 per cent gamma benzene hexachloride cream (Lorexane) repeated after a week or 25 per cent monosulfiram lotion (Tetmosol lotion) diluted with 3 parts water to 1 part lotion and applied 2 or 3 times. These treatments are highly effective but reinfestation is common if any close infected contact is overlooked. In a heavy institutional outbreak, monosulfiram soap (Tetmosol soap) may be brought into general use throughout the period and provides good protection for attendant staff. Although it may be desirable to change and launder all clothing and bedding, this is not strictly necessary as the residual skin applications will kill any wandering mites.

9 Lice infestation

Lice are exclusively human insect parasites which flourish in cold or temperate climates where personal and hair cleanliness is neglected and clothing seldom changed. Lice and scabies thrive in similar conditions and the two infestations may be found in the same patient.

Head lice (*Pediculus humanus* var. *capitis*) are the most common variety and affect about 10 per cent of school children in Britain. Body lice (*Pediculus humanus* var. *corporis*) are a closely related variety but are uncommon in ordinary civilian conditions. They occur amongst vagrants and may become common in military groups and in prisons and were formerly important vectors of typhus (*Rickettsia prowazeki*) and relapsing fever (*Borrelia recurrentis*). Crab lice (*Phthirus pubis*) are less common and live only on the pubic hair, being spread by venereal contact. Adult lice deposit eggs which are firmly attached to hair or textile fibres. The eggs (nits) survive for about a month and appear as woolly grey granules attached to individual hairs. Lice feed by biting the skin and a raised itching papule forms at the site. Scratching quickly results in secondary infection with pustule and scab formation.

In individual patients lice are readily destroyed by the application of 1 per cent gamma benzene hexachloride cream or 0·5 per cent malathion scalp application, but reinfection is common unless all members of a family or group are treated simultaneously and there is a permanent improvement in hygiene.

Emergency treatment of large numbers of soldiers or prisoners for body lice consists of the insufflation of 10 per cent DDT in talc inside the clothing.

CHAPTER 39

Pyrexia of Uncertain Origin (PUO)

The majority of patients who present with fever are suffering from benign self-limiting viral infections lasting on average 2–4 days. These often present with respiratory symptoms such as sore throat and cough and occasionally with gastro-intestinal symptoms. However, the high probability of a benign illness is not a good reason for making a snap diagnosis of 'flu' or 'gastric flu' without a proper clinical assessment of the patient. This all too often leads to mistakes and delays which could be avoided by adequate history taking (including contact with infection, foreign travel, animal contacts and the drinking of raw milk) and by physical examination. In pyrexial illness the situation may change rapidly, so that clinical reassessment is important if new symptoms develop or if the fever persists. This systematic assessment of fever cases will help to develop an awareness of the symptoms, signs and situations which are indicative of more serious disease, requiring urgent hospital investigation. In the absence of alarming features the persistence of fever for more than one week tends to be labelled as PUO and deserves full investigation.

In the majority of pyrexial cases the cause will be infection and it is therefore desirable for such patients to be investigated in isolation conditions, this being particularly important in the case of patients who have recently returned from foreign travel.

The assessment of a case of PUO may be difficult because the possible causes are too numerous to review at one time.

The following classification breaks down the possible causes into more manageable groups and is not intended to be exhaustive.

1 Generalized infections
Tuberculosis—primary, pulmonary, miliary, pleural, meningeal, renal, abdominal, bone and cryptogenic.

Glandular fever
Typhoid and paratyphoid
Brucellosis
Septicaemia
Toxoplasmosis
Q fever
Mycoplasma infection
Psittacosis
Cytomegalovirus infections
Leptospirosis
Malaria
Amoebiasis
Miscellaneous viral infections

2   Localized infections

Nervous system	meningitis, brain or spinal abscess, sinus thrombophlebitis
Respiratory system	otitis media, nasal sinusitis, pneumonia, lung abscess, pleurisy
Cardiovascular system	subacute bacterial endocarditis, deep vein thrombophlebitis
Alimentary system	cholecystitis, cholangitis, liver abscess, subphrenic abscess, pelvic abscess
Genito-urinary system	urinary infection, perinephric abscess, uterine sepsis
Musculo-skeletal system	septic arthritis, osteitis

3   Collagen, auto-immune and allergic diseases

Rheumatic fever
Rheumatoid disease
Periarteritis nodosa
Systemic lupus erythematosis
Dermatomyositis
Systemic sclerosis
Crohn's disease
Drug-induced fever

4   Malignant diseases

Hodgkin's disease; other lymphoma group
Leukaemia
Carcinoma lung, kidney, bowel, etc.

Investigations

The following are some of the more important investigations which may need to be carried out.

Haemoglobin, white cell count and ESR
Throat swab
Sputum cultures
Blood cultures
Faeces cultures
Urine microscopy and culture
Tuberculin test
Paul–Bunnell
Widal
Brucella agglutination
Toxoplasma dye test
Viral cultures and antibodies
Chlamydial, mycoplasma and Q fever antibodies
Leptospiral antibodies
Amoebic serology
Cerebrospinal fluid examination
Chest X-ray
Abdomen—straight X-ray
Nasal sinus X-ray
Blood film for parasites
Faeces for parasites
Plasma protein and electrophoresis
Rheumatoid factor
Anti-nuclear factor
Anti-streptolysin 'O' titre

Cold-agglutinin titre
Liver function tests
Pyelogram
Cholecystogram
Barium meal and enema

Radioactive scan—liver, brain
Bone marrow examination
Biopsy—liver, lymph gland

CHAPTER 40

Hospital Infection

Infection is one of the major hazards of hospital practice in spite of present-day high standards of hygiene, antisepsis and asepsis.

Some outbreaks of infection are caused by the admission of a case or a carrier of a communicable disease, such as salmonellosis or infantile gastroenteritis. In this respect, hospitals are no different from other closed institutions with communal sleeping, eating and toilet arrangements. Any ward may be involved but surgical, geriatric, maternity and children's units are at a greater risk than the others. Long-stay mental hospitals are subject to recurrent outbreaks of gastrointestinal infections such as dysentery, because of the difficulty in maintaining satisfactory personal hygiene with uncooperative patients. The position might be improved by the admission of all suspicious cases (including patients with diarrhoea and fever or with a recent history of these symptoms) to isolation. Consideration might also be given to the bacteriological screening of all patients admitted to the more vulnerable units, for example, faeces culture on women due to enter maternity units.

In the event of an outbreak, affected wards are closed, the transfer of patients is only allowed for the most urgent reasons, cases are isolated, staff and patients are screened for the carrier state and, when empty, the wards are thoroughly cleaned and disinfected before readmitting patients.

A further problem in hospital is the effect of opportunist micro-organisms on a highly vulnerable patient population. The factors responsible for this situation include the following:

1 The intensive use of antibiotics in hospital encourages the emergence and increases the population of antibiotic resistant organisms by the process of selection. This happens mostly with staphylococcal and coliform species which tend to be more pathogenic than unselected organisms and are obviously more difficult to treat. There also tends to be an increase in naturally resistant organisms such as *Pseudomonas* and *Proteus* species.

These resistant organisms may cause infections which reach local epidemic proportions at times. Measures to control such outbreaks include the isolation of cases, a search for carriers, the cleaning and disinfecting of wards and operating theatres, and, in the more severe outbreaks, the closure of wards. The intensive use of antibiotics rarely helps to control outbreaks; in fact, more success has followed the severe restriction or the complete withdrawal of antibiotics.

2 Hospitals include vulnerable age groups (the newborn, young children and the elderly) and sick people of all ages who are less able to withstand the effects of even mild infections.

3 Many hospital procedures and techniques increase the susceptibility or facilitate the entry of infection, including the following:

(*a*) *Injections.* These may lead to local infections, the most serious of which is gas gangrene. Syringes contaminated with infected blood may spread hepatitis B. The use of disposable individual syringes has reduced this problem.

(*b*) *Intravenous infusions.* These may lead to septicaemia (commonly staphylococcal or coliform) from infection at the site of entry or rarely from contaminated intravenous fluids. The risk of septicaemia increases with the duration of the intravenous drip, so this is kept to a minimum. Intravenous fluid should not be used if the contents show the least cloudiness. Any addition to infusion bottles should be carried out under strict aseptic conditions.

(*c*) *Instrumentation.* The passage of instruments in an infected urinary or biliary tract may lead to a severe septicaemia usually with coliform organisms and frequently complicated by endotoxic shock. Appropriate antibiotic treatment does not relieve the shock and may even temporarily aggravate it, by increasing the production of endotoxin as the organisms are killed. Treatment to relieve the shock includes the use of corticosteroids and intravenous plasma. Prophylactic antibiotics used before such instrumentation should be considered.

(*d*) *Surgical operations.* Wound infections occur (usually staphylococcal, coliform or even clostridial) and these may lead to local spread or septicaemic infection.

In certain circumstances the use of pre-operative prophylactic antibiotics may be helpful; e.g. the use of metronidazole before intestinal surgery to reduce the risk of bacteroides infections and the use of penicillin before limb amputation to reduce the risk of clostridial infections.

(*f*) *Immunosuppressive drugs and corticosteroids.* These increase the susceptibility to infection and serious generalized infections may occur with many types of normally harmless organisms. The tendency to infection is also increased in other conditions which interfere with immunity such as leukaemia or other reticulosis. Chickenpox is a specific hazard to all these patients. Any unexplained pyrexia or general deterioration in such a patient should be fully investigated for infection.

(*g*) *Renal dialysis and haemophilia.* Units for these cases are susceptible to dangerous outbreaks of hepatitis B.

(*h*) *Organ transplantation.* These patients incur the hazards of disturbed immunity, and are prone to unusual infections including fulminating cytomegalovirus infection.

There are further details of some of these conditions in the appropriate chapters (Viral Hepatitis; Streptococcal Infections; Staphylococcal Infections; Gastroenteritis of Infancy; Clostridial Infections).

CHAPTER 41

Chemotherapy

The rational use of antibacterial drugs requires a sound knowledge of the possible bacterial causes of the various infective conditions. There are no consistent principles governing the use of antibiotics but the following points are noteworthy:

1 The isolation of a pathogenic organism from a healthy person is not always an indication for antibiotic treatment.

2 Acute diarrhoeal disease is rarely helped and may be seriously aggravated by 'blind' or repeated courses of antibiotics.

3 Most of the sore throats and upper respiratory tract infections in children and adults are viral in origin. These infections are self-limiting and in normal circumstances antibiotic treatment is neither necessary nor helpful. Exceptions, where antibiotics may play a useful role, are streptococcal throat infection, a child prone to recurrent otitis media following throat infections, the patient with a history of rheumatic fever and the chronic bronchitic prone to secondary chest infection following viral upper respiratory infections.

Local antibiotic preparations such as lozenges have no value in the treatment of mouth and throat infections and may cause painful mucosal superinfections.

4 Persistent pyrexial illness, without immediately alarming symptoms or signs, requires full investigation and a diagnosis before antibiotics are given. Otherwise drugs given for no definite reason will almost certainly have no definite effect and the clinical picture and diagnosis may be obscured and delayed. An exception is the planned therapeutic test which may provide diagnostic information by the response to the drug. Examples include the use of antituberculous drugs in very prolonged pyrexia and metronidazole in febrile hepatitis.

5 A single antibiotic is generally adequate for most purposes but antibiotic combinations are necessary in:

(i) tuberculosis, to prevent the emergence of bacterial resistance;

(ii) bacterial endocarditis and septicaemia, to enhance therapeutic activity;

(iii) life-threatening infections of unknown aetiology, often septicaemic or affecting the respiratory tract. Such cases require
immediate intensive antibiotic treatment with combinations of
drugs capable of countering the more likely organisms, as soon
as the necessary laboratory specimens such as blood cultures
have been collected;
(iv) mixed infections.

Combinations of bactericidal and bacteriostatic drugs should
be avoided because of the possibility of antagonism, though this
is rarely a problem in clinical practice. In certain conditions,
bactericidal drugs are to be preferred over bacteriostatic drugs.
The latter group depend on the body's normal defence mechanisms for the final elimination of the organisms and such
defences may be faulty in bacterial endocarditis, severe septicaemic states and in patients with defective immunity.

6 Resistant strains of micro-organisms emerge in direct proportion to the use of antibiotics, particularly in hospitals, so
that the drugs should always be used with discrimination.
Bacterial resistance may develop in different ways. In some
species a tiny minority of naturally resistant bacteria gradually
replace the sensitive strains. Other species develop the ability to
excrete the enzyme beta-lactamase which inactivates the penicillins and related antibiotics. Intestinal bacteria are able to
convey multiple antibiotic resistance within their own and in
related species by the transfer of resistance-carrying plasmids.
This mechanism continues to operate even in the absence of
exposure to antibiotics.

7 Antibiotic prophylaxis is generally valueless except in the
prevention of:
(i) bacterial endocarditis in patients with heart disease undergoing dental treatment;
(ii) recurrent attacks of rheumatic fever;
(iii) wound infection following bowel surgery;
(iv) gas gangrene in thigh amputation for obliterative arterial
disease;
(v) meningococcal infection in contacts;
(vi) whooping cough in infants who are home contacts.

8 Antibiotics in renal failure:
(i) drugs such as erythromycin, clindamycin and fucidin, are
excreted largely by extra-renal mechanisms, so that no precautions are necessary;

(ii) the penicillin group of drugs, though excreted via the kidneys, are relatively non-toxic and require only minor modification of dose;

(iii) drugs such as gentamicin, kanamycin and cephaloridine require careful monitoring of peak and trough serum levels to achieve the full therapeutic effect without toxic effects.

Table 11 summarizes the normal dosage and common toxic effects of the more commonly used antimicrobial drugs. With some drugs (including the penicillins) a greatly increased dose may be used by intravenous infusion (IV) in severe or difficult infections and these are also indicated in Table 11.

TABLE 11   Antimicrobial drugs for systemic use

Drug	Route given	Adult dose	Child dose	Toxic effects
Benzylpenicillin	IM	0·5–2·0 mega units 6-hourly	0·5–1·0 mega units 6-hourly	(a) Anaphylaxis (b) Rash and fever
	IV	24–48 mega units/day		Rarely, tubular damage and haemolytic anaemia in high doses
Penicillin V	Oral	250–500 mg 6-hourly	25 mg/kg/day	As benzyl-penicillin
Ampicillin	Oral/IM	500 mg–1 g 6-hourly	40 mg/kg/day	As benzyl-penicillin (Rashes common)
	IV	10–20 g/day	250 mg/kg/day	
Amoxycillin	Oral	250 mg 8-hourly	10–20 mg/kg/day	As Ampicillin
	IM/IV		10–20 mg/kg/day	
Cloxacillin	Oral/IM	250 mg–1G 6-hourly	25 mg/kg/day	As benzyl-penicillin
Flucloxacillin	Oral/IM	250 mg–1G 6-hourly	25 mg/kg/day	As benzyl-penicillin
Carbenicillin	IM	1–2G 6-hourly	50–100 mg/kg/day	
	IV	20–30 g per day	250–400 mg/kg/day	Electrolyte overload
Carfecillin	Oral	500 mg–1G 8-hourly	30–60 mg/kg/day	As benzyl-penicillin

TABLE 11 (*contd.*)   Antimicrobial drugs for systemic use

Drug	Route given	Adult dose	Child dose	Toxic effects
Cephaloridine	IM	500 mg–1G 6-hourly	30–60 mg/kg/day	(a) Rashes (b) Anaphylaxis
	IV	4–6 g/day	60 mg/kg/day	(c) Nephrotoxic (d) Cross-allergenicity with penicillins
Cephalexin	Oral	500 mg–1G 6-hourly	25–50 mg/kg/day	(a) Intestinal upset (b) Rashes (c) Cross-allergenicity with penicillin
Streptomycin				
(a) General use	IM	500 mg–1G 8-hourly	25 mg/kg/day	Ototoxic Rash Drug fever
(b) Antituber-culous	IM	1G daily	10–20 mg/kg/day	
Isoniazid	Oral	200–300 mg/day	5–10 mg/kg/day	Neurotoxic Liver damage Antagonizes phenytoin
Sodium Amino-Salicylate	Oral	10–15 g/day	300 mg/kg/day	(a) GI tract upsets (b) Rash and fever (c) Jaundice
Ethambutol	Oral	15 mg/kg/day		Optic neuropathy
Rifampicin	Oral	600 mg/day	15 mg/kg/day	Liver damage Antagonizes birth control pill
Tetracycline	Oral	250–500 mg 6-hourly	25 mg/kg/day	(a) Diarrhoea (b) Bone and teeth damage (infancy)
Chloramphenicol	Oral/IM	250 mg–1G 6-hourly	40 mg/kg/day	(a) Diarrhoea (b) Aplastic anaemia
	IV			(c) Grey syndrome in neonates

TABLE 11 (*contd.*)   Antimicrobial drugs for systemic use

Drug	Route given	Adult dose	Child dose	Toxic effects
Erythromycin	Oral	250–500 mg 6-hourly	25 mg/kg/day	Jaundice
	IM		25 mg/kg/day	
Fusidic acid	Oral	500 mg–1G 8-hourly	25 mg/kg/day	
	IV	1·5–2G per day	20 mg/kg/day	
Clindamycin	Oral	150–300 mg 6-hourly	10–20 mg/kg/day	Diarrhoea Pseudo-membranous colitis
	IM/IV	300–600 mg 6–8-hourly	15–40 mg/kg/day	
Kanamycin	Oral	500 mg–1G 6-hourly	40 mg/kg/day	Not absorbed
	IM	1G daily	10–20 mg/kg/day	(a) Nephrotoxic (b) Ototoxic
Colistin	Oral	2 mega units 6-hourly	100,000 units per kg/day	Not absorbed
	IM	0·75–1·5 mega units 6-hourly	50,000–100,000 units/kg/day	Mildly neurotoxic and nephrotoxic
Gentamicin	IM	80 mg 8-hourly	1 mg/kg 8-hourly	(a) Ototoxic (b) Nephrotoxic
Neomycin	Oral	500 mg–1G 6-hourly	40 mg/kg/day	Not absorbed
Amikacin	IM	15 mg/kg/day in 2 equally divided doses	15 mg/kg/day in 2 equally divided doses	As gentamicin
Sulphonamide	Oral/IM	1G 6-hourly	50 mg/kg/day	(a) Rash and fever (b) Marrow depression (c) Crystalluria
Co-trimoxazole (tablet or 5 ml amp contains:	Oral	2–6 tablets per day	1–4 tablets per day	
Trimethoprim 80 mg Sulphamethoxazole 400 mgm)	IM/IV	10 ml twice daily	Equivalent of 6 mg trimethoprim per kg per day	(a) As sulphon-amides (b) Megalo-blastic anaemia

TABLE 11 (*contd.*)   Antimicrobial drugs for systemic use

Drug	Route given	Adult dose	Child dose	Toxic effects
Nalidixic acid	Oral	1G 6-hourly	50 mg/kg/day	(a) Intestinal upset (b) Neurotoxic (c) Photo-sensitivity (d) Haemolytic anaemia
Metronidazole	Oral (200 mgm tab) IV	1–4 tablets 3 times a day 500 mgm 3 times a day	$\frac{1}{2}$–2 tablets 3 times a day	(a) Gastro-intestinal symptoms (b) Rarely, neutropaenia and parasthesiae (c) Avoid alcohol

Index